M000216645

CHEMICAL
INSENSITIVITY

How The Environment Cost Me My Life:
My Struggle with Multiple Chemical Sensitivity

by Sandy Major

SJMCS LLC

*It was Sandy's wish that any net proceeds from
the sale of this book be donated to charitable
organizations dedicated to research into
MCS. It is our intent to honor her wishes.*

Publisher: SJMCS LLC

www.sjmcsllc.com

Copyright 2021 Sandy Major

Second printing

This book is copyright under the Berne Convention.

All rights reserved.

No Reproduction without permission.
Printed in the United States of America

ISBN: 978-1-0879-8814-6

CATALOGING INFORMATION:

Major, Sandy

CHEMICAL *IN*SENSITIVITY

HOW THE ENVIRONMENT COST ME MY LIFE: MY
STRUGGLE WITH MULTIPLE CHEMICAL SENSITIVITY

Table of Contents

Acknowledgements

I appreciate all who have contributed so much to this ever-expanding effort to clarify and stamp out this debilitating illness.

I especially want to thank John, my husband, for reviewing, editing and keeping the project moving.

John's big brother and sister-in-law, Jim and Joan Major, are especially appreciated for all the time they spent editing and correcting drafts of the book. Jim is an accomplished author himself, and I am so grateful for his and Joan's input.

My sister Laura and her husband, Joe Bird, have provided wonderful comfort and support during these weeks. Joe's research and suggestions for the book were, I believe, sent by God.

I am grateful to my sister-in-law Linda Brown, who suffered from MCS long before I knew what the initials stood for. I especially thank Linda for sharing her own personal experiences with MCS and for her contributions to this book.

I also want to thank my children, siblings, and other family members for trying to understand my situation over the years. I so much regretted all the times we were not able to be together, and all the hassles involved in the few times we were able to spend time together.

Sandy

Timeline

August 2001
We buy our Tybee condo

December 2003
We move into newly constructed home on Tybee

July 2011
Lake Tahoe wedding – first "exposure" to MCS

June 2012
We move into newly remodeled home on Tybee

October 2013
Tiki torch party gives early warning of MCS

October 2016
Hurricane Matthew hits Tybee
First evacuation to Western North Carolina

September 2017
Hurricane Irma hits Tybee
Second evacuation to Western North Carolina

November 2017
Begin short-term lease in Tryon

April–May 2018
Purchase lot in Tryon foothills
Sign Blue Ridge Log Cabin contract
Begin new home construction

September 2018
Initial cancer diagnosis

October 2018
Move into new mountain home

November 2018
Surgery

September 2019
Cancer returns

December 2019–February 2020
I write this book

Chapter 1

IN THE HOSPITAL

It was November 19, 2018 – Thanksgiving week – and I found myself lying on a hospital gurney, waiting to be wheeled down the hall into the operating room that was waiting for me. My surgeon was holding my hand and praying that his hands would receive divine guidance as he opened me up and attempted to remove all the invasive cancer cells that had brought me to this place and time.

I liked that.

The praying, not the surgery.

My husband, John, a retired businessperson, and I had gotten up early that morning. I had packed a half dozen reusable grocery bags with things I thought I could eat, wear, and safely have around me following my surgery. I had even brought my own small air purifier in hopes of being able to somehow improve the atmosphere in the small room I would occupy for the next unknown number of days.

1

I had felt pretty good over the past few weeks and had experienced an unusually high level of energy. John and I had met with landscapers to talk about how to best improve the lot on which our beautiful new log home stands. Just last night, we had stayed up late, hanging pictures throughout our new house. There was so much to be done as we began this new chapter in our lives.

And yet, at this point in the hospital, I thought I was ready for God to take me if that was His will. But in the year since my surgery, I have learned that God still had some work for me to do before I left this earth.

It had been four years since John and I had celebrated our 50th anniversary at the beach on Tybee Island, Georgia, surrounded by our two wonderful

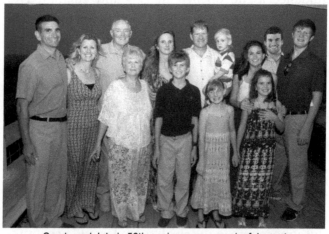

Sandy and John's 50th anniversary was a joyful event celebrated with friends and family on Tybee Island. Sandy and John pictured with their children and grandchildren.

children and their seven equally wonderful children. Friends and family gathered on this special day to be with us and to wish us many more years together. It was shortly after that anniversary celebration that my life began to change in a way I could never have imagined.

In the pages that follow, I hope to share with you what the work that God had planned for me has turned out to be and, more importantly, the string of events that brought me to this place, on this day, in Thanksgiving week, 2018. And I will share with you events and circumstances from my own five-year personal nightmare.

That nightmare has a name. It is called Multiple Chemical Sensitivity, a condition brought about by things that you touch, eat, smell, and otherwise experience every day of your life.

You may not be aware that you live in a toxic environment that is hidden right in front of you, all around you, everywhere you go. This environment cannot always be avoided, but there are things you can do to improve your own personal chances.

You will learn, as I have, that while I am chemically sensitive, much of the world around me is chemically *insensitive.*

I honestly believe that God has inspired me to put these words on paper while I am able to, and that you will read them.

While you still can.

3

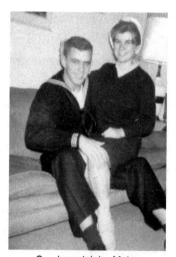

Sandy and John Major

Chapter 2
WHO AM I AND WHY AM I WRITING THIS MEMOIR?

To understand the conditions and circumstances that brought me to this point in my life, you need a little background about me.

My name is Sandy Major. I grew up in Georgia and Michigan, and I met John, my husband, our freshman year at Michigan State University in 1963. We married the next year. Now, almost 56 years later, our two children have blessed us, collectively, with seven grandchildren.

Both of our children were born while John was serving his two tours of duty in Vietnam with the United States Navy. Much of my working life was spent in the Pittsburgh area, where I founded a childcare center that remains successful today. I later relocated to Western Maryland, where I helped to design and start up a small business incubator building and program, which continues to flourish today.

In 1997, after a small business counselor conference in Savannah introduced me to Tybee Island, we began annual vacations to this small barrier island paradise.

Throughout my adult life, I have been active in local business, church, civic organizations, and even local politics. Getting involved and doing my part to better the places where we lived, and to improve conditions for those around me have always been important to me.

In addition to my career activities, I partnered with my husband in our own small business. Our careers took us to Pittsburgh, Western Maryland, and Tybee Island, Georgia.

In 2001 we purchased our first property on Tybee. Although our consulting business was still going strong, we thought that we had found the place where we would spend our retirement years together.

You will learn much about what happened since as you read the pages of this book.

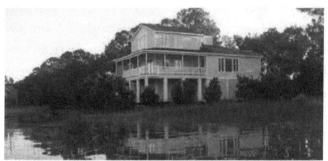

Sandy and John's first home on Tybee – their "big house" on the tidal creek. They thought they would be there forever.

Chapter 3

MULTIPLE CHEMICAL SENSITIVITY – WHAT IS IT AND WHY SHOULD YOU CARE?

To help you understand what I, and my family, have experienced over the past five years, let me tell you about this thing known as Multiple Chemical Sensitivity (MCS).

My reasons for writing this book were not to try to discover the cause of MCS, or determine if it is a true "disease" or illness in medical jargon. I am not qualified to do that. While my life experiences with MCS are real and painful, it is not scientific evidence as understood by the medical profession. My sincere hope is that this book can serve as a companion to other people who suffer from MCS, and perhaps give them resources to minimize the condition's effects on their lives while offering my own anecdotal evidence and life experiences to these pages. I pray that these words will help others understand the difficulties faced by sufferers, and enable non-sufferers to appreciate this little-known condition. Stated simply, I want to support, in words and spirit, those who suffer, and to open the minds and spirits of those who don't so that they might understand this condition.

If you read the medical literature on MCS, you will find more questions than answers. Some have said its origins are psychological or psychosomatic. Others claim that it is an immunological disorder with neurological symptoms. One more recent scientific article suggests that normal brain and neurological function is altered when chemical exposure triggers the production of too much of a certain neurotransmitter called N-methyl-D-aspartate. It is a poor transmitter of neurological messages. This chemical interferes with normal function by, in a manner of speaking, cutting in front of the normal brain function neurotransmitter, Glutamine, in receptor cells. [1]

The result is interference with neurological messaging. It is as if the brain loses its "cellphone" signal and ability to make a call due to the triggering effect. Whether this trigger is written in your genetic code or is something acquired or learned due to chemical exposure is still unknown. The more research that is being conducted, the more it has become clear that not only are the symptoms and suffering real, but that there is likely a physiological cause that might someday be treatable. One significant study, Women with Multiple Chemical Sensitivity

Have Increased Harm Avoidance and Reduced 5-HT1A Receptor Binding Potential in the Anterior Cingulate and Amygdala, published on line January 22, 2013, at PLoS One, 2013; 8(1); 2013, suggests changes in the serotonin cycle could be responsible for increasing the human avoidance instinct to foul odors that correlate to things that are dangerous to humans. How the serotonin cycle is changed in MCS sufferers is not understood, nor is it known if the altered serotonin cycle is a precursor that makes a person prone to MCS.

I don't have the answer. Perhaps it is glutamate injections or supplements. Perhaps it is serotonin therapy of some sort. More brain chemistry studies seem to hold the answer and perhaps a cure.

A recent short article from Johns Hopkins, published on their HEALTH web page under the title Multiple Chemical Sensitivity, concludes:

At this time, it is a controversial issue as to whether it is a clinical diagnosis or not. Many in the medical community lean towards these symptoms being physical manifestations of psychiatric illness rather than a primary medical illness while others in the medical community, along with organizations agree that multiple chemical sensitivity is a negative physical reaction to certain chemicals. There is debate as to whether multiple chemical sensitivity should be classified and diagnosed as an illness.[2]

Perhaps it is something else altogether.

9

My own experience follows the common pattern of an acute chemical exposure experience leading into MCS. It is complicated, and perhaps commingled with my cancer diagnosis. I have come to believe that MCS is likely the human body's warning system – a warning from the effects of chemical exposure gone haywire.

Think of it like a car alarm that has gone off because the door handle was bumped, but that now cannot be turned off. The sound of the alarm is with you constantly, with some relief in the form of a lower volume at times.

When someone learns that a friend or family member has cancer, they pretty much understand, at some level, what that means. Surgery, chemotherapy, radiation, hair loss, and hopefully, prayerfully, someday remission and resumption of normal activities.

Not so with Multiple Chemical Sensitivity, the condition my family learned about at Lake Tahoe and which later came to fill my waking and even sleeping moments. You will learn more about our Lake Tahoe experience as you continue to read.

Google MCS and you will find that the medical community cannot agree on what it is, what causes it, or even if it's real, although I'm sure the millions of people who suffer from some degree of MCS will testify to its "realness." Topics that pop up in response to your search will include "MCS – is it real?" You will learn that some in the medical field consider MCS to be "idiopathic" – that's a condition that arises "spontaneously" or with no known cause.

To me, that's something of a cop-out. I do not think my condition arose spontaneously but rather as a result of continuous exposure to a variety of terrible, toxic chemicals. Some of these were purchased by me out of a lack of understanding of their toxicity, while others were forced on me by Mother Nature and human efforts to clean up behind her.

When I look on the Internet to try to determine how widespread this affliction is, I find a wide range of reported percentages of the population.

A 2018 study[3] of MCS by Anne Steinemann, Professor of Civil Engineering and Chair of Sustainable Cities from the University of Melbourne School of Engineering, was published in the *Journal of Occupational and Environmental Medicine.* In it she defined MCS as a medical condition characterized by adverse health effects from exposure to common chemicals and pollutants, from products such as pesticides, chemical odors from new carpet and paint, renovation materials, diesel exhaust, cleaning supplies, perfume, scented laundry products, and air fresheners. MCS can cause a range of acute, chronic, multi-organ, and disabling health effects, such as headaches, dizziness, cognitive impairment, breathing difficulties, heart palpitations, nausea, mucous membrane irritation, and asthma attacks.

11

Professor Steinemann found that the number of people in the United States who had been diagnosed with MCS had increased by 300 percent over the past 10 years. This increase, according to the study, while "astonishing," is not unexpected, due to our daily use of toxic products.

The study further found that 12.8 percent of our population has been medically diagnosed with MCS, and 25.9 percent – more than one out of every four people in our country – reported chemical sensitivity. Of that 25.9 percent, 86.2 percent have had related health problems when exposed to consumer products with fragrances. They have had to avoid public places where they might be exposed, or have missed work because of an unfriendly environment at the workplace.

Other reports call those of us with this affliction "human canaries" which relates to a mining tradition dating back to 1911, in which miners brought canaries into coal mines to test the air for carbon monoxide or other toxic gases that could hurt humans. If the canaries started to die, the miners knew the air was turning toxic.

Millions of Americans suffering from MCS are telling us that the canaries are dying.

Unfortunately, dying canaries have very little power against the huge lobbying efforts in our nation's capital by the industries that produce the poisons that we all breathe, and to which some of us just have a stronger reaction.

Different people will react to different toxic chemicals in different ways, but we all will experience some of the symptoms such as: headache, fatigue, dizziness, nausea, congestion, itching, sneezing, sore throat, chest pain, changes in heart rhythm, breathing problems, coughing spasms, muscle pain or stiffness, skin rash, diarrhea, bloating, gas, confusion, trouble concentrating, memory problems, and mood changes.

I have personally experienced most of these symptoms in various settings. One particular incident stands fresh in my mind. Each year, for about a decade, John and I would drive to either Charleston or Jacksonville and connect flights to St. Thomas and

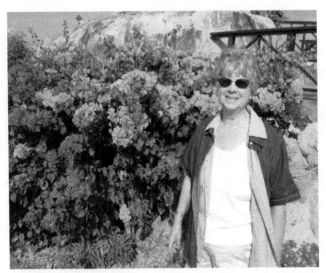

Between the fresh Caribbean air, the ocean and the wonderful people, Sandy found that the British Virgin Islands gave her a "happy place."

the British Virgin Islands. During one such adventure, after I had begun experiencing MCS, we had selected a hotel near the airport where we could catch our originating flight in the early morning. I had only to walk into the room to know that my requests for special cleaning and laundry, which were sometimes respected, had been ignored. I immediately began having many of these symptoms. I was dizzy, confused, and my mood became desperate as I looked around for a way to escape. Although the hotel was ultimately able to find a less-offensive room, our trip had proven to be off to a very uncomfortable beginning. When you look at the range of reactions that can be brought on by the things we voluntarily introduce into our environment, you can understand the reaction that so many of us have.

When we lived on Tybee Island, both John and I were very active in our community and in our church. When I began experiencing reactions to the inevitable hugging and handshaking at every Sunday's worship service, I found I could no longer attend.

John explained to our pastor why I wasn't coming and told him that as much as 10 percent of the U.S. population suffers from MCS to some degree. The pastor was astonished, and said "You mean that as many as 40 people sitting in our congregation every Sunday are reacting to those around them?"

John's response was, "No. They're all at home."

Our church made an effort to create a "fragrance-free zone" that consisted of two rows of chairs at the back of the sanctuary properly labeled and asking anyone wearing any kind of fragrance to sit somewhere else.

What we found was that when the seats were all taken, as they usually were thanks to God and inspired teaching from the pulpit, there would be empty seats in the rear and those seats would be taken by latecomers – fragrances or not. Being close to the door and allowing a quick and unseen early exit was a bonus, so the seats were always taken by latecomers, warning signs notwithstanding.

The ushers, doing their duties of administering communion and passing the collection plate, also found the seats in the back very handy for their needs and, unfortunately, some of them seemed to be walking advertisements for after-shave.

Through this book I hope to share my personal experiences with those who may not be aware of what our environment may be doing to them and their families, and some suggestions on how to avoid it.

In the appendices, I will provide tips and suggestions for those who have not yet begun to experience the negative effects our environment is having on them.

I call one of the appendices "What Can I Do to Protect Myself and Those Around Me?" I hope that through the information provided here, both from my own experiences and from those of others, I am able to reach and alert some potential sufferers and that they are able to choose a healthier path for their own lives.

I cannot say definitively that my own MCS was directly or indirectly accountable for my later diagnosis of cancer. I can say, without hesitation or doubt, that because of this condition, treatments that are embraced by conventional medicine have been denied to me.

My oncologist suggested that I undergo the chemical and radiation therapy that my family doctor, who has an excellent grasp of alternative methods and chemical sensitivity, says will kill me.

MCS is real.

It was so distressing to learn that I am afflicted with MCS. It was far more distressing to realize that so much of the world around me is afflicted with chemical *in*sensitivity.

We live in a nation where we instinctively trust the manufacturers of the products that surround us every day. We trust them when they tell us that their products are safe.

We trust that our government is strong enough and smart enough to see through lobbying efforts and protect us from any product that could be harmful to us "when used as directed."

But then I think about asbestos, talcum powder,

pesticides, weed killers – things we can and do buy only to find out later that class action lawsuits have been initiated because people are dying from them.

My own experience tells me that the only "treatment" for this condition is to avoid exposure to the toxins that cause the reactions. So far, the world that produces those toxic products has not shown much interest in promoting their avoidance.

I wonder why?

If my story can help anyone avoid the triggers of MCS, better endure it or better understand someone who suffers, I will have achieved my goal. With each person helped or made to appreciate living with this disorder, my spirit will burn brighter.

References:

[1] Dr. Jill Carnahan, Multiple Chemical Sensitivity, August 10, 2018 blog on environmental toxicity.

[2] https://www.hopkinsmedicine.org/health/conditions-and-diseases/multiple-chemical-sensitivity

[3] Anne Steinemann, Ph.D., "National Prevalence and Effects of Multiple Chemical Sensitivities," *Journal of Occupational and Environmental Medicine 60,* no. 3 (March 2018): e152-e156.

Chapter 4
A WEDDING AT LAKE TAHOE AND LEARNING ABOUT MCS

As the surgeon is finishing up his prayer, we join in a very sincere, especially on my part, "Amen." So be it! As I laid there on the gurney, I remember thinking about when and how I first became aware of Multiple Chemical Sensitivity. I didn't realize that as I was reading about this terrible affliction, I was actually getting a glimpse into my own future.

My brother David and his wife, Linda – more from her later – had graduated from high school in Michigan, packed their car and trailer with all their earthly belongings, and headed west.

Way west. All the way to South Lake Tahoe, California.

In the years since, we had visited them once, and we had been able to otherwise connect in person only a couple of times. We had no idea what Linda had been going through. Due to personal medical circumstances with their youngest son, they had decided that David would stay at home and provide the needed care. Linda would work to provide the family income and benefits.

The personal sacrifices that have been required of this couple, even seen from such a distance, have been an inspiration for all of our family members. The added challenge presented by Linda's MCS has made their response to their circumstances even more remarkable.

In the summer of 2011, their oldest son was to be married. His bride-to-be turned out to be a local television talent who came from a well-to-do Lake Tahoe family, so a wedding to be remembered was planned.

To our surprise, several months before we were scheduled to fly to Reno and drive to Lake Tahoe, we received this letter from Linda, the mother of the groom-to-be:

Dear Family & Dear Friends,

I am so very much looking forward to seeing all of you! My enthusiasm is only tempered somewhat by the letter that I must write, but here goes:

Many of you are aware that I am sensitive to perfumes, and many of you are not aware of the extent of my hypersensitivity. I had a tough year in 2010 (transitional migraines), and I remain on medication and unfortunately remain even more sensitive to perfumes. In plain words, they disable me. The only recommended action for those like me is to avoid perfume, which brings me to the reason for this letter. I respectfully ask that you review the personal products that you use, and to please refrain from using some of them during your visit, and prepare by purchasing non-scented or lightly scented products for your visit with us.

I know this will be a hassle, and I am so sorry, but please believe me, I would not ask you to do this unless I felt I had to. My intention is to ward off the worst symptoms of disabling migraines and disabling sinus headaches during this very exciting time. Unfortunately, Nathan (our disabled son) also suffers from this affliction, and his headaches border on the unbearable. I will list products that we use and which will not cause a reaction in us. If you have specific products that you feel you cannot do without, or you think are only very mildly scented, I would be happy to give them the sniff test in a nearby store; just give me the details and I will get back to you. (This all might sound perfectly ridiculous, but it is the reality for those of us chemically sensitive to perfume and living in a world which is essentially toxic to us.) Here are the details:

All personal care products are suspect because they are all routinely scented. Other than perfume and aftershave, the most highly scented products are those for the laundry, men's deodorant, and all lotions. Listed below are the products that we use or can tolerate:

21

(Note: to avoid confusion for the reader, this list was updated by Linda in 2020)

Perfume & Aftershave:

None – please launder clothing, which may have residual scent.

Laundry products:

Their scents are made to last, so please launder all clothes you will be packing with one of these products:
Any non-scented laundry detergent
or Biokleen Free & Clear
Laundry Liquid (plant based)
Bounce free & gentle dryer sheets

Deodorants:

Dove Sensitive antiperspirant
Sure unscented antiperspirant & deodorant (has a light scent)
Acure fragrance free

Lotions:

Griffin Remedy Body Lotion Unscented
CeraVe Moisturizing Lotion Fragrance Free

Facial:

Olay Fragrance Free or Sensitive Skin products with or without sunscreen
Neutrogena Healthy Defense Fragrance Free or Sensitive Skin products

Sunblock:

Neutrogena Sensitive Skin

Sunscreen Fragrance Free

Soaps & Body Wash:

Cetaphil Ultra Gentle Body Wash Fragrance Free

Everyone Soap unscented

ShiKai Shower Gel unscented

Facial:

Neutrogena ultra-gentle Hydrating

Cleanser fragrance free

CeraVe Hydrating Cleanser

Shampoos:

Free & Clear Shampoo for Sensitive

Skin /Conditioner also available

It truly pains me to ask that you go through all
these extra efforts. All I can do is **thank you**,
and I do – from the bottom of my heart!

——Linda

Like I said, we were surprised to receive this letter
since our awareness of Linda's issues was superficial,
at best. Only relatives and close friends of the groom,
therefore those who would be in closest physical
contact with Linda, were asked to alter their routines.

We had a hard time imagining that such a
large event, with possibly hundreds of people in
attendance, could be successfully pulled off with such
strict fragrance requirements.

It was.

Most of the activities were conducted outdoors – easy to do in California in the summertime – and those that were inside were held in airy, well-ventilated spaces. As far as we could tell, there were no flagrant fragrant violations, and the wedding came off as an event we all will cherish and remember forever.

I was now aware of this thing that was out there, but I was not aware of the impact it would, in about four years, have on my life and how I would be forced to deal with it.

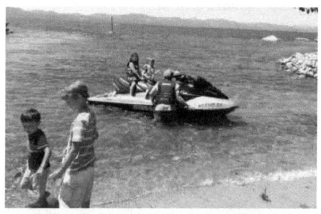

A family wedding in Lake Tahoe was an incredible time with loved ones and the first real exposure to the horrors of MCS.

Chapter 5
LINDA B'S STORY

My first exposure, literally, to MCS was in planning for our nephew's wedding at Lake Tahoe. My sister-in-law, Linda B, the mother of the groom, introduced me to the condition as we prepared for her son's Tahoe wedding.

I have asked her to share her story with us, and what follows is in her own (first person) words:

* * *

I had virtually lost my health in 1995 and was diagnosed with Chronic Fatigue Immune Dysfunction Syndrome (CFIDS), currently known as Myalgic Encephalomyelitis. I met all the symptom criteria for the illness, which still does not have a recommended treatment, let alone a cure. I was unable to work full-time for a year but felt I wasn't essentially over CFIDS until four years later. It was at that time that I took a closer look at the hypersensitivity I had been experiencing with perfumes and its relationship to my health.

In reviewing my experience with CFIDS and my memories of the signs that signaled the beginning of my continuing problems when exposed to scents and current health issues, I am absolutely convinced that the "chemical sensitivity" to perfumed products came first. I will explain.

I am and have been for many years hypersensitive or extremely allergic to "perfumed products" (which I will refer to simply as perfumes or scents). This includes most personal products (colognes, scented laundry products, soaps, deodorants, lotions, sunscreens, etc.) and other airborne scented products, such as dishwasher soaps and furniture polish. The scents in these products have a petroleum base, and I am also very sensitive to other petroleum-based products, such as some plastics, and some high-gloss magazines and catalogs. I also have reactions to diesel fuel and chain oils. The (petroleum) oils in all of the scented products are what helps to distribute long-lasting scents into the environment and, therefore, what I believe is causing my reactions and health issues.

Allergies* often develop after multiple exposures to the offending agent(s). It is not surprising that one could develop a serious allergy or reactions to petroleum products, which are toxic and so pervasive in our society. I am not suggesting that one can treat a chemical sensitivity to perfume as they would an allergy – it is commonly thought that avoidance is the only option for those affected. My sensitivity was left unacknowledged and untreated at the time of my CFIDS illness, and the built-up toxicity caused me to virtually lose my health.

There are clear signs and memories that I was reacting to perfume prior to my CFIDS diagnosis. Had I known what was happening, I am sure that I would have many more examples, but what follows is what I can attest to. I experienced my first migraine in my thirties. It was a "classic" migraine with visual disturbances, and so it was clearly defined as a migraine. I cannot remember what my age was at the time, but I remember my doctor stating that it was "unusual to get one's first migraine after age 30." I also remember that perfume and a bright light were present when I got the visual symptoms preceding that first headache. This may have been the start of perfumes triggering reactions in me, and I began to get a couple of migraines every year. My strange and deteriorating health symptoms began when I was in my late 30s. I remember one significant incident prior to my health crash and my CFIDS diagnosis. I had a little product left in my perfume bottle, and when I put it on, I thought that it smelled different and may be "going bad." Although I tried to wipe it off, I received a compliment on its scent that evening. Was this also a sign that my relationship/reactions with perfume had changed? I am sure that it was the last time I wore perfume. While attending a women's group meeting within that first year after the CFIDS diagnosis, I was unable to concentrate during a meditation because an incense stick was burning, which I had to extinguish. It's ironic that the first person I met with perfume sensitivities was a member in that women's group (apparently she was not at the meeting mentioned above). In spite of that, I clearly did not understand the symptoms or consider that it could also be my underlying problem.

It became apparent to me at about the same time I recovered from CFIDS (four years after my diagnosis) that all perfumes were affecting me – not just the overbearing scents. I asked for accommodation at work, and a voluntary scent ban was requested from co-workers in the building. This was of some help but also led to further ostracizing by a number of people who did not understand or care to understand.

The most compelling reason I have for believing that my chemical sensitivity preceded my CFIDS was that once I had recovered from the illness, I recognized that a longer duration of low-level exposure to perfume triggered the same CFIDS symptoms in me. This happened repeatedly. I would feel as if I had flu-like CFIDS symptoms for days without any stomach upset – just a general feeling of unwellness and exhaustion.

So what symptoms do I get from perfume

exposure? Immediate reactions can include burning sinuses, congestion, upset stomach, an inability to think and speak clearly, migraine, post-nasal drip, coughing, and light-headedness. I can have anxiety, serious mood swings (mostly sadness or anger, but I can also feel suicidal), and I have more difficulty sleeping. I even had heart palpitations from one co-worker's laundry product. I have had reactions to perfumes for a minimum of 25 years, and probably closer to 30. My symptoms have worsened through the years, and later-onset symptoms have included occasional shortness of breath, burning and seriously congested lungs, and (undiagnosed) asthma. I have learned that asthma can be immediate/acute, and delayed (secondary or late phase), and may include nighttime and cough-variant asthma. (This list only includes asthma types that I have experienced.)

It seems odd that I could have such severe reactions to perfume for years and not be aware that perfumes were the cause of them. I believe that is due to the fact that I did not start out with this problem, and so I did not suspect it – compounded by the fact that scents are so prevalent in our environment that it is hard to separate them from our world. I was unaware that my reactions to perfume could be delayed (other than when an individual wearing a very strong scent would trigger a migraine). For instance, my "brain fog" reaction might follow someone visiting

29

and exiting my office by 10 or 20 minutes. This is also compounded by being diagnosed with an illness that received some credibility from the CDC.

Many people do not think of perfumes as being toxic. They smell good, right? How can they be bad for you? It is because the perfume industry is largely unregulated – the product formulas are considered secret and proprietary. The U.S. government, as per their published report, is aware that many people have issues with perfume, and some have serious problems, but fragrance is neither a food product nor medicine and has not been taken seriously. It is time for a change. Besides the standard way to deliver drugs (by pill or injection), it is quite common to deliver medications through the skin via patches, and to spray medicines and vaccines via the nasal passages. Our air is being polluted, and chemicals are being delivered to us without our permission. We should be outraged!

The Depth and Breadth of the Problem

Perfume has taken its toll on me. My reactions continue to escalate, and its damage has continued to accumulate. I needed to work, and I had exposure to perfume almost every day. I had allergy shots for 20 years to take the load off my immune system. Approximately a decade ago, I got into a "daily migraine syndrome" pattern and have needed to take antihistamine daily ever since. Five years ago,

I noticed some wheezing from my upper lungs. I was given the all-clear by a pulmonologist but, unfortunately, that was not correct. Approximately six months after retirement, I was diagnosed with moderate COPD caused by emphysema. I am sure it was caused by perfume exposure. Since COPD is the third leading cause of death in the U.S., per the American Lung Association, it will likely be the cause of my death.

Perfume is not a safe product, and the number of people affected may be growing. I have met many of them. I asked my employer to keep their voluntary scent ban active after my retirement, because 30 percent (15 of 50) of those using the building regularly had shared their sensitivity stories with me (from instant headaches, to vomiting after exposure). Perfume sensitivities often run in families, and my own son has had some extreme migraines after exposures. When people are ill and as they age, they become more prone to its negative effects. I worry that the rise in childhood autism may be due to perfume toxicity. Our homes are full of scents – laundry products, dishwasher and dish soaps, cleaning and polishing products, hair products, lotions, etc. – and they transfer to our furniture and virtually all our possessions. My body and mind are often overloaded or overstimulated by scents – wouldn't children also be affected? I recently met a young father who claimed that his 3-year-old autistic child was doing so much better after they removed scents from their home. The people I know or have met who have problems with scents, other than the ones I mentioned above include: two hairdressers and the daughter of one, my dental hygienist, four doctors I frequent, my former allergist, two friends with perfume-induced asthma, relatives of two of my former co-workers, a title specialist, a woman I met who was looking for a good unscented facial moisturizer while I was also, a woman who was holding a scarf to her face as I entered an elevator, a woman I sat next to at a seminar, and most recently one of Sandy's three younger sisters, Laura. These people are everywhere but seldom stand out. I have known or bumped into so many people afflicted with this illness, it makes you wonder how many millions have the problem.

Sandy is my sister-in-law, and we have more in common than this illness and her brother. We are intelligent, accomplished, compassionate, and giving souls who raised beautiful people and touched many others. We helped build our dreams with our long-term, supportive spouses. I can assure you that Sandy wants to live out her luscious, golden years with her wonderful husband of more than 55 years, but she is dying because her chemical sensitivity kept her from the treatment she desperately needed. This is a great tragedy for her and for so many families who feel totally devastated by her prognosis. Sandy has fought to get the word out to help others who suffer with this affliction (and may not even know they have it). I can carry some hope that the progressive medical field can prolong my life from the damage caused by perfume, but Sandy is losing her fight, and her hope lies with and for you. Let us hope that she will be a catalyst to make real and lasting change.

There is nothing inherently wrong with scents. They can improve your mood, calm, energize, make you happy, boost your confidence, and leave a lasting (hopefully pleasant) impression on others. Yet, perfume sensitivity greatly reduces quality of life for a great many, takes people's health, and creates isolation for those affected and their loved ones. It shortens lives and steals quality years. What is the answer? Manufacturers must become more responsible. The public does not need scents that go on for days, and laundry products that can last three months. The last perfumed product I had was a vanilla scent that had a castor oil base – it was plenty powerful. Let's keep the petroleum products and chemicals out of perfumes! The public needs to be informed and demand safety. Let there be awareness and movement towards responsible wearers. Smoking was banned from many public places. It's a start towards healthy air that we can all breathe and enjoy.

Let's hope that the perfume industry takes the toxins out of scented products, and that using heavy scent becomes very unpopular.

*Allergies differ from chemical sensitivities in that allergy triggers IgE-mediated inflammation, whereas chemical sensitivity alters TA1 cells and chemical antibody levels. The term allergy is used here because I and probably most people have a general understanding of its meaning. For further information about chemical sensitivity visit: www.ncbi.nlm.nih.gov/books/NBK234795

Chapter 6
Tybee Tiki Torches and Discovering My Own MCS

When we first moved to Tybee Island, Georgia, in 2003 after purchasing our rental condo, we decided to buy a lot and build our dream home. Surrounded by the salt marshes, a beautiful home with nearly 5,000 square feet (including the garage) gave us everything we ever thought we would need. Our small business consulting company was going strong, so John was traveling quite a bit. During construction, we were able to rent and stay in what we called our "beach shack" – not very pretty but special in its own way.

A few years after moving into our new home, we were able to purchase what we called our "little house," directly across the street. Partnering with our builder, this small creekside home served us well as a short-term rental for six years. Then one day in 2012, I said to John, "Let's sell this big house and move across the street into the little house." So we met with our partner, negotiated a purchase price to buy him out, and planned the total remodeling of our "little house." A second story master bedroom/bathroom was added as well as a general update of the main floor.

Although I wasn't aware at the time, the construction activities – tearing down and building back up – proved to be filled with toxic chemicals that were having an effect on me.

The little house was old, having first been constructed as a barracks for training Navy divers in the 1940s and later moved to its present location. In

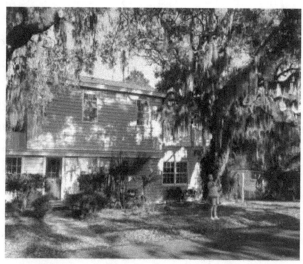

Plans were drawn up to sell the big house and move into the little house across the street, which would be gutted and rebuilt. Remodeling complete, the move to the little house was accomplished.

our remodels, we did lots of things wrong, including covering much of the home with carpeting.

Shortly after we sold the big house and moved across the street, we held a party for friends behind the house, next to our boat dock and the tidal marsh. We had propane grills cooking hotdogs and hamburgers and, to light the night, we had purchased about a dozen tiki torches, fueled by that kerosene-like fuel that, although I didn't realize what was happening at the time, proved to be one of my main triggers.

This was the first of many miserable nights I would spend, itching, having trouble breathing, at times feeling dizzy and having to retire from the group early.

It was not to be the last.

I could only wonder what was going on as I found myself tearing up, struggling for breath, and feeling an overall sense that I was being invaded by some unknown force.

Before long, I would find out.

CHAPTER 7

FAILING EYESIGHT AND CATARACT SURGERY THAT WASN'T TO BE

Multiple Chemical Sensitivity was to have a profound life-changing effect on every aspect of my existence.

During the summer of 2015, John and I both became aware that we were developing cataracts in both eyes and needed surgery.

We had, for some time, been patients of some of the finest eye doctors through the Georgia Eye facilities in Savannah. John was able to go through the preparation and surgery for both eyes and his cataract surgery was completed.

I, on the other hand, along with my ever-present MCS, was to learn that in order to have this surgery, I would be exposed to products and chemicals that would make it impossible for me to tolerate the surgery.

I did my best to seek out non-chemical alternatives that I could tolerate but, even with assistance from this excellent institution, I was unable to find anything that would allow me to go through with the surgery.

As a result, at this stage of my life, I am unable to sit in the bright sunlight, watching all the beauty that surrounds me in our amazing North Carolina mountain home. If the sun is shining and I have to be somewhere, driving myself is out of the question. I am forced to sit in the passenger seat, dark glasses in place, scarf wrapped around my face, a mask pulled over my eyes, and a hat pulled down over the mask and scarf in order to tolerate even the most modest of bright days.

At home, I long for cloudy days and nighttime, when the bright rays of the North Carolina sun no longer torture me, and I am able to enjoy my home without wearing sunglasses inside with all the blinds

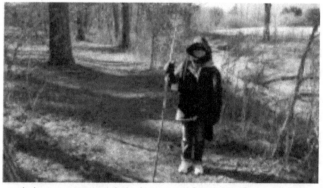

In her ever-present dark glasses and floppy hat, Sandy had a number of favorite places to walk in the Polk County area.

drawn. Even then, I must have the dimmest of artificial lights, causing others in the room to sometimes resort to flashlights to find what they are looking for.

Because of this severe light sensitivity, I am dictating the chapters of this book, because I am unable to stare at the screen of my computer.

I cannot say with certainty that MCS is directly responsible for my failing eyesight, and my inability to address and correct the problem, but I feel sure that there is a link. Without MCS, I feel confident that I, too, could have successfully completed the cataract surgery that would have allowed my eyesight to serve me today.

I pray that people who have not yet begun to experience this condition realize that it could be stalking them already, and that they learn and practice everything that can be done to ward it off as long as possible.

Chapter 8

Hurricane Matthew – Our First Evacuation from Tybee

As I think back over the times and events that brought me to this point in my life, the massive storm that scraped the Georgia coast in October of 2016 stands out.

Our first property on Tybee Island, Georgia, purchased in 2001, was a beautiful oceanfront condo that we turned into a vacation rental. This property proved to be especially popular with tourists during the summer months, which, unfortunately, is also the peak of hurricane season.

Year after year, we would tell our prospective renters, "Don't worry about hurricanes." You see, there's this thing called the Georgia bight, where the land takes a giant bend to the west so the hurricanes can blow right past us. This was good for us, but not so good for the Carolinas. We weren't misleading renters; we actually believed it.

We knew that back in 1893 Tybee had been ravaged by one of the worst hurricanes in U.S. history. That was a long time ago and nothing like that had happened since.

But this approaching hurricane seemed different. On several occasions over the past 15 years, when storms appeared to be aiming our way, John would be checking the Weather Channel constantly. Each time he would suggest that we might want to seek higher ground. I would try to calm him down and say, don't worry about it. We will be safe. Remember the Georgia bight.

Not this time.

Something was telling me that it was time to go. This storm, now a category 5 hurricane pounding the Caribbean islands, would be one that Tybee folks would talk about for a long time.

So, we secured our boat, tied down everything that could be moved by the wind, packed Rowdy the cat in his cage, and headed north.

Our daughter owns a vacation rental property in North Carolina, so evacuating to that area was a logical path of retreat for us. Unfortunately, her home was rented to someone else, so we found another short-term rental in the same area.

As we sat in our cozy log cabin, enjoying the warmth and the calm, we watched Matthew on television take the unusual path of churning up Florida's Atlantic coast. It didn't make a direct hit but kept chopping up everything in its way. Matthew stayed just far enough offshore to maintain its speed but close enough to leave a path of destruction as it made its way north – directly toward Tybee.

How weird it seemed, watching folks from the various weather reports standing on our familiar beaches while the wind behind them picked up and relocated awnings, street signs, and anything not securely tied down.

This was the storm that we had been saying we would never see. While not nearly as terrible as the last major storm to hit Tybee, Matthew would indeed bring its own blend of wind, rain, and surge.

The Tybee Mayor issued a mandatory evacuation order shortly after we left. Predictably, the traffic heading west on Tybee's only road off the island became snarled. Hurricane-force winds were soon recorded at the Tybee lighthouse.

The Mayor called Matthew the worst storm the island had seen in more than 100 years. When residents were finally allowed back to their homes, the *Atlanta Journal Constitution* reported:

...they found an obstacle course of shingles, siding and palm fronds along the main drag; whole neighborhoods and roads, particularly on the island's south side, under water for long stretches of time; a dozen homes or condos without roofs; and industrial-sized coolers, power poles and lines and old railroad ties deposited on the roads in ungainly fashion by the ferocious winds that tore through this town of 3,000 residents.

We owned the vacant lot across the street from our house. More than a dozen large pine trees had shaded this lot, but no more. All of our pines were now laying horizontally in a pattern that extended to our neighbors' driveway which was now completely blocked. This was the case all over the island.

When we returned to our home, we found our yard – front and back – buried in about a foot of "wrack" (mostly dead marsh grass and other debris) delivered to us by the rising waters from the marsh and left behind by the receding tide.

Others were not so lucky. All we had in front of our house were sawed-up pine trees and piles of dead marsh grass. On the next street east of us nearly every home had been flooded. In the days following the storm, yards became staging places, waiting for pickup, not only for trees and yard debris, but for furniture and appliances, ripped out wallboard and pulled up floors, all of which had been destroyed by the rising waters of Hurricane Matthew.

For me, the worst was coming, when the sun came out, the winds died down and the waters pulled back. Now the massive job of cleaning it all up began.

Residents with trees downed by the storm were told by the city to cut them into four-foot pieces and leave them by the side of the road for pickup. For several weeks we were serenaded from early in the morning until late at night by the sound of hundreds of chain saws preparing the dead trees for the trucks that were to come.

Chain saws run on gasoline, one of my prime triggering agents. I was virtually unable to leave the house because of the pollution.

Then, even before the chain saws were done with their necessary but noxious duties, the trucks came. Imagine giant dump-style trucks with grappling hooks on swivels designed to pick up the tree carcasses and pile them in the truck. Imagine the atmospheric cocktail resulting from fumes from the chainsaw gasoline mixed with those from diesel fuel from the trucks, and you will have imagined what we were living with following the storm.

The parking lot of one of Tybee's favorite restaurants was used as a staging ground for all the tree pieces. Piles of these reached 30 feet and higher as they waited to be chipped and shipped somewhere else. More equipment. More gasoline. More reaction from me.

Meanwhile, the fresh air and beauty of the North Carolina foothills had planted its seed with us.

And it was beginning to grow.

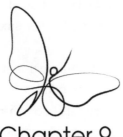

Chapter 9

DOCTOR C – MY NATUROPATHIC ANGEL

After we moved into the little house across the street, I knew I was "in it," meaning this condition I've come to know as MCS. In addition to the move, I'm sure the overall Savannah air quality contributed as well. Within six months of making the move, I remember thinking: "This place is making me sick."

All I knew at the time was that I was chemically sensitive. I knew I couldn't be around people with fragrances. I knew I couldn't handle gasoline, propane or anything like that. I had met with many doctors over the years, including conventional medical doctors and allergists. But it wasn't until 2017, when I met with Dr. C in Savannah, that it all came together for me. I had learned that a Naturopathic doctor, such as Dr. C, treats the whole body, using natural, sometimes ancient remedies. He was able, through questioning and testing, to show me the things that I was reacting to. These included:

- As a child, playing near a coal storage area
- Stripping and refinishing furniture over the years
- Spending a lot of time around older people who smoked, even though I never smoked a cigarette in my life
- Stripping the paint off an old fireplace using a toxic product and an electric grinder
- Having gasoline splash back on me while refueling and being unable to change clothes for some time
- Using ammonia products to remove bathroom mold
- Walking barefoot at the "little house" on an upstairs porch that had been covered and sealed with caustic roofing products
- Being around toxic building products through multiple new builds and re-builds

Dr. C said it's like having a glass that you keep adding more and more water to until it eventually overflows. I learned that experts call that the "rain barrel effect." And that's what my body did after so many years of being exposed, even as a child, to so many toxic chemicals; my body finally overflowed after moving into the little house across the street.

Dr. C is a Naturopath and is the only doctor up to that point in my life who had been able to help me understand what I am experiencing, and how to make some improvements. He recommended a specific detox program for me, and I was able to implement the program over a three-month period shortly after we had made our initial move to North Carolina.

When I finished the "boot camp" program, in the spring of 2018, I felt really good.

The program recommended by Dr. C was a combination of eating organic foods, walking about a mile a day, swimming, kayaking – that kind of thing – and colonics. I also took IV's, mostly vitamins and glutathione. My treatments included castor oil packs and oatmeal and magnesium baths along with hot and cold therapy.

Discovering Dr. C made so many things clear that had been mysteries to me. I will forever be grateful for the time I spent with my Naturopathic Angel.

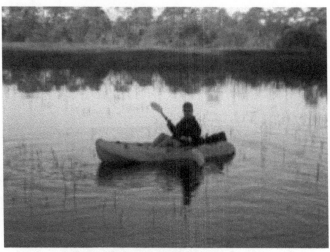

Sandy loved kayaking, whether on Tybee
or on the lake in North Carolina.

Chapter 10
HURRICANE IRMA BLOWS US
AWAY FROM TYBEE

It was unusual to have the opportunity to spend time with John, just the two of us in my small hospital room while I was fighting desperately to regain enough strength to go home. Although the hospital was only about an hour from our new home, I found out right after surgery that it was also worlds away in terms of having an environment that I could tolerate. I had been moved to a small private room on a typical ward where the nurses and staff do their best to satisfy the needs of all their patients. Patients who summon them throughout the day and night. Because of the activities and noises going on around the clock, neither I, in my hospital bed, nor John, in his little chair next to my bed, got much sleep. This gave us time to talk and reflect on the events that had brought us here, to Western North Carolina.

September 11, 2001, will always conjure up images of terrible destruction for Americans. But for many who live on the east coast, the date, in addition to the memories from the attack on our country, will now bring about thoughts of another 9-11.

Before Matthew, Georgia's east coast had managed to go more than a century without serious damage from a hurricane. It was easy to think that Tybee wouldn't be hit for another hundred years or so.

But Mother Nature had other plans for us. For the second time in less than a year, Tybee was to be ravaged by an Atlantic storm, this time Hurricane Irma. Irma tore into Florida as a major category 4 hurricane on September 10 and headed north, toward the Georgia coast.

While Matthew had been, for us, mainly a strong wind event, Irma had slowed down considerably before Tybee would feel its impact. This time flooding was the major problem.

Tragically, many of the folks in low-lying areas of Tybee, who were just recovering from their losses after Matthew, found themselves again ripping up floors and carpets and placing their furniture and appliances on the curb for pickup.

Just a few days before Irma reached Tybee, we had traveled over to Wilmington, North Carolina, to spend Labor Day with our daughter and her family. From our beachside hotel, we watched with increasing concern as Irma made its way northward toward the east coast of the U.S.

By the time we said our goodbyes to family and headed back toward Tybee, we had decided that we would once again heed the evacuation order, which at that time was still voluntary.

That would change.

So, once again, we tied down and packed up. Rowdy was back in his cage as we headed back to Western North Carolina, a place that was beginning to symbolize, for us anyhow, safety and refuge from the storm. This time, our first rental in Tryon turned out to be a disaster. While I had, as I always do, requested a property that had been cleaned with fragrance-free products, this one had not been. In addition to the strong odors from harsh cleaning products, the small cottage had problems of its own – rotted wood in the windowsills, electric extension cords stretched across the floor, and a general musty smell that I couldn't handle.

In spite of the fact that the rental agency was unwilling to make any kind of adjustment, we knew we wouldn't be able to stay. So after one torturous night, we grabbed our gear and our cat and moved on.

I honestly believe this was meant to be. Good fortune and God's hand led us to a beautiful little apartment in nearby Landrum, South Carolina. This

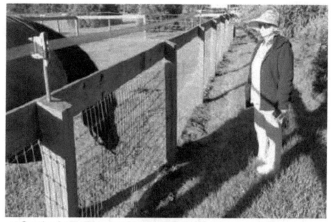

Sandy chats with one of her new friends at the equestrian ranch
where she and John evacuated for the second hurricane.

place was amazing – located on top of a horse stable,
which was part of an equestrian ranch.

The memories we gathered during our week at
this wonderful place will be with us forever: walking
around the fenced areas with the horses following
us, and big, friendly ranch dogs always there to
greet us. Our stay there was truly a once-in-a-lifetime
adventure.

It might seem strange that I am so sensitive to
artificial smells and fragrances and have such dramatic
reactions to such toxic products but was able, not
only to tolerate, but actually delight in the strong
smells that inevitably associate with horses, barns, and
dogs. My experience tells me that the environment
found in stables and paddocks is natural and, while

sometimes unpleasant, creates an entirely different reaction in me. I was fine. I was better than fine in this natural environment, surrounded by nature and able to breathe without any difficulty at all.

Meanwhile, Irma was flooding Tybee. Again, we sat in the Carolina foothills, far away and safe from the rising waters, and watched our neighbors being hammered by this storm.

When we left our temporary ranch home, we knew that at least part of our future would be in this area. We were thinking we could spend our summers here and winters back on Tybee.

That's what we were thinking in September of 2017.

Chapter 11
OUR FIRST YEAR IN NORTH CAROLINA:
FINDING A HOME

So much has happened since our two evacuations from Tybee Island, which brought us to Western North Carolina. After Hurricane Irma brought the worst flooding event in over a century, we were sure we wanted to spend at least part of the year away from that small barrier island in the Atlantic Ocean. And to us, "away" had come to mean the mountains and foothills of Western North Carolina.

John had been serving on Tybee's City Council. His term expired after the last meeting in December 2017, and he would not be seeking another.

The morning after that final meeting, we packed up everything we could and headed north. I had found a small log cabin we could rent on a short-term basis, and we signed a six-month lease, expiring at the end of May 2018. We later extended that lease until November.

Other than the fact that we couldn't drink the water and the HVAC system was more than twenty years old and not very efficient in cold weather, the cabin was delightful. Situated near the top of one of the area's mountain roads, the

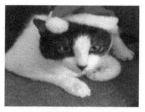

In the small rental cabin, while a new home solution was being sought, Rowdy was into the Christmas spirit.

cabin was a short walk from a beautiful waterfall and summertime views of acres and acres of one of the area's most prolific crops – kudzu.

Very shortly after our return to Western North Carolina, the decision was finalized: we would not be looking for a summer home away from Tybee, but a full-time, permanent residence in the foothills. This decision would involve our divesting ourselves of our Tybee properties: a rental condo, our home, and a vacant lot across the street.

My younger sister was staying in our Tybee home while we searched for a new home in North Carolina and was able to keep an eye on that property in our absence.

During that summer, 2018, as we looked for a local physician, we found Dr. B, who was establishing a family practice in a nearby community and working through the local hospital while her new offices were being prepared.

She totally understands MCS. In addition to being an M.D., she also appreciates and works with all kinds of alternative and integrative approaches, and is more interested in reducing prescription dependency than on increasing one's medications. She was perfect for us. After initially practicing as a conventional M.D., she had retrained to become an integrative doctor, partnering with her patients as they work together to find the best combination of life activities to improve their health.

When her new offices opened in April 2018, John and I were her first patients. Following one of our early visits to her office, John and I were looking for a place to walk and happened by a much-used mountain trail nearby. As I stepped out of the car, I saw several dozen beautiful butterflies congregating on the ground.

With John's phone-camera rolling, I stepped into the group and lifted my arms as they swarmed around me. The back cover picture for this book came from that special event and remains one of my all-time favorite photos.

What we had anticipated being a fairly easy process of finding a place to live turned out to be much more of a challenge. Homes that might have been ideal were found to fall short of our requirements in one way or another: appliances in the basement, carpeting with their accompanying fragrance issues, propane cooking or fireplace – I couldn't even go inside. There always seemed to be something that said to us "this won't work."

As we continued to explore Polk County and its surrounding areas – some of the most beautiful places we had ever seen – we realized more and more that we were being called to look into log cabins. After our building experiences in Maryland and Tybee, especially our last project, remodeling the "little house," we thought we would never undertake another construction project. But everything we looked at kept telling us that a log cabin would meet our needs. Everything could be on one level. No propane or carpeting. A special fireplace. No toxic off-gases.

When we visited the model homes at Blue Ridge Log Cabins, we knew this was what we were being called to do. Blue Ridge manufactures their cabins indoors, in an assembly line process. There are no fragrances, and we could have the layout exactly as we wanted. Our home would be delivered to our lot (which we didn't yet have) in four "boxes" that would look like a home at the end of the first day. Great news from a fragrance standpoint, not so good from a timing standpoint, as our search for a lot for our new home got serious.

So now that our new home was getting built, we needed a place to put it. John T, our realtor who had so patiently shown us so many homes over the past three months, continued to work even harder looking for a lot. Finally, in February 2018, we decided on a lakeside lot on the other side of Melrose Mountain from our rental.

We were excited, not only about the lot but about everything this community had to offer: lakes for swimming, kayaking and fishing, private roads for walking, and breathtaking views of the Western North Carolina mountains.

We met with a couple of builders recommended by Blue Ridge and chose one. He and the excavator met with us to verify the feasibility of the lot – all of this while our home was being built in Campobello, South Carolina. With the help of Blue Ridge's Don O and their staff, we were able to pick out our fixtures, appliances, and other details that would be included with the home on delivery day.

As we moved toward the end of 2018, we were very excited about our new home and the time we would have to share in it.

The trip from our rental cabin to our building site was only about twenty minutes. As property owners, we had full access to our new community's roads, lakes, and other amenities. That summer, during construction, we took full advantage of everything our new community had to offer. We had brought our kayaks up from Tybee and could regularly be seen using them or swimming or just hanging out at the lake, which was directly across from our new home site.

Our Certificate of Occupancy was issued on October 24, 2018, and we were excited about moving in. Arrangements were made to have the new furniture we had purchased delivered as well as all our "stuff" from storage. As we were preparing for our move, I was diagnosed with cancer.

It's hard to explain the mixed emotions we both were feeling. The joy and anticipation of moving into an incredible new home to almost immediately facing the biggest challenge we had ever experienced was daunting, to say the least.

The move went smoothly, but as we settled in, the upcoming trip to the hospital and my surgery hung over everything we did.

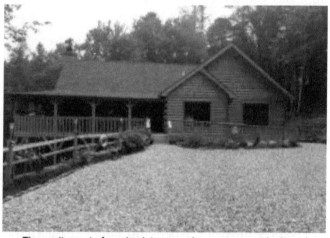

The excitement of moving into a new home was overshadowed by Sandy's cancer surgery, which was only a few weeks away.

Chapter 12

SMALL ROOM, SMALL CHAIR, AND TOXIC STAFF: TRYING TO SURVIVE IN A TOXIC ENVIRONMENT

I remember reciting Psalm 23 – my favorite verse from scripture – over and over in my head, as unseen hands and faces moved my gurney from my prep room into the operating room.

The Lord is my shepherd; I shall not want.
He maketh me to lie down in green pastures.
He leadeth me beside the still waters...

Hours later, when I finally woke up, I felt my freedom had been taken from me. Even if I had been able to move on my own, I was locked into my bed, my legs held in position, vibrating to avoid clotting.

I remember feeling like a baby. I couldn't turn over. I couldn't drink anything despite a burning thirst.

I looked around at what was to be my home for the next unknown number of days – days that in retrospect were among the most terrible four days of my life.

My primary care physician had written an introductory letter to the hospital, explaining in detail my MCS condition and cautioning against anyone coming into my room with any kind of fragrance on their person. I thought the letter would get the attention of the hospital staff. Here is an excerpt from the body of the letter:

To whom it may concern:

Sandra Major is my patient and has multiple chemical sensitivities. She will be bringing her own sheets, blanket, pillow, and if possible HEPA air filter to plug into the room. She is very sensitive to cleaning chemicals, to inhaled odors, so we request her room not have any new furniture or carpet, air fresheners, new plastics, latex or alcohol cleaners used prior to her entrance. She is at increased risk of adverse reactions to anesthesia as a result of her chemical sensitivities. She also needs to bring her own post-op food such as homemade bone broth and liquids such as green tea. She cannot have sprite or any drinks with food colorings or corn syrup added. No solid foods with dyes or additives. Medications need to be dye- and filler-free as much as possible. Hospital staff cannot wear any perfumes or aftershave, nor have cigarette smell on their clothing. Please flag her chart as an MCS (multiple chemical sensitivity) patient.

I soon found out that the letter had not been shared with any of the staff.

It seemed the doctors and nurses understood my situation and I never felt invaded by any of them. Other staff, including food service and certified nursing assistant's (CNAs), were another story, and we were unable to ward off their frequent invasions.

One of the nurses finally posted a very clear notice on my door, clearly stating that anyone with any fragrances on them must not enter, but it went unheeded.

I will always remember the nurse who told me: "You don't go to a hospital to get well."

Hand sanitizer dispensers were everywhere, and anyone entering the room would use them. I know they were there to protect me, but instead were triggering my old familiar MCS responses.

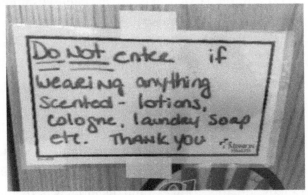

Despite a letter from Sandy's doctor and a sign placed on the door by a nurse, invasions by staff wearing fragrances were constant in the hospital.

John had checked into a local hotel and had thoughts of spending his late evenings there. We soon realized that he would be living and sleeping in the small, uncomfortable chair that was jammed between my bed and the wall, coming to my rescue every time a fragrance-laden staffer came in for one reason or another.

If we were able to get some time between fragrance attacks, we would most likely have our peace interrupted by the very frequent nurse calls from other patients. The piercing alarm, set off by someone needing help, would continue until answered. And that could and often did take a long time.

It's encouraging to find on-line that some major hospitals have adopted policies to outlaw fragrances on the premises. The U.S. Centers for Disease Control and Prevention (CDC) sets an excellent example with its own extensive policy which, according to the website https://invisibledisabilities.org/environmental-illness/cdc-fragrance-free-policy/ has been in place since 2009. Other institutions should follow this example.

The policy clearly defines what is meant by scents and fragrances and to instruct what is to be done in the event of an infraction. I am hopeful that all hospitals, doctors' offices, and facilities where the public gathers will eventually adopt similar policies.

My surgery had been on Monday. Thursday was Thanksgiving day, and while I am sure I wasn't ready to be checked out, we insisted and headed home. Because of my early departure from the hospital, I left with the need of using a catheter. This later led to other horror stories, but I was excited to be returning to our wonderful home in the mountains.

I was never so happy as when we were driving up our driveway and seeing our log cabin waiting for us.

Homecoming was quiet, but all I wanted was to get into my own bed. I spent quite a bit of time there over the next few weeks, confined by my catheter and immobility.

We had the foresight to purchase a walker, and after a while I was able to transit the halls on our hardwood floors and could sit up in our great room.

John was learning to prepare meals and otherwise do the basics of taking care of us both. It was weeks before I began to have any sense of normal, and by then we had made several trips to visit my primary care doctor, the surgeon, and my oncologist. This was very draining, both physically and emotionally, and the entire process was much harder than I had expected. Every time we would make one of these trips, I would always be very happy to be back in my own home when we were done.

Chapter 13
My Christmas Angel – So Much Help in So Many Ways

We had moved into our new home in late October 2018, and my surgery was less than a month later, on November 19th. After my surgery, I realized that I was too emotional to talk to anyone, especially those family members that I loved most of all, and this lasted for several months. But the day after we got home from the hospital, we had a welcome surprise. Cassandra, who had been so helpful to us in our rental cabin, as well as through all the packing and unpacking from our move, showed up unannounced with a dish of Shepherd's pie. I was only able to eat the potatoes on top of the pie, and John enjoyed the rest.

We feel so fortunate to have had Cassandra in our lives. I have seldom known such an energetic, focused, and hardworking young person. She comes from a large Mennonite family and is the only girl in the midst of brothers. In addition to her cleaning business, she was also serving customers at a local coffee shop, starting her day on the 6 a.m. shift.

Cassandra was always looking for ways to better herself, whether it be through some training program or through starting a new business. I am confident that she will continue to be successful and bring her special light into the lives of those she touches.

Back when we were making our plans to transition from our little rented cabin to our new mountain home, we knew we would need help. A neighbor we had met recommended Cassandra, and we soon had her working in the small cabin, helping with all the activities that would ensure that we left it in better condition than we had found it. We were so impressed with how she was able to clean the outsides of windows that were 6 feet off the ground by opening the window, sitting on the ledge and leaning out.

When we made the move, she again proved invaluable, not only with the construction cleaning, but with all the packing, unpacking, and putting away of all our earthly belongings, some from the small cabin and some from storage.

Over this past year, a year of so many dark challenges, Cassandra has been such a shining star in my life.

To me, because she was such a regular and welcome presence during all the activities involved with our move, and because so many of the most difficult times happened during the Christmas season of 2018, that is why I think of Cassandra as my Christmas angel.

Chapter 14

Our Second Year in North Carolina
Living a Dream in the Middle of
a Nightmare

Following my abbreviated hospital stay, made shorter than planned by my constant exposure to toxic fragrances, we returned to our new home, and I began my recovery.

This was Thanksgiving day, and we were trying (to paraphrase 1st Thessalonians 5:18, NIV) to be "joyful and praise God *in* all things" even if we could not be "joyful and praise God *for* all things."

One of my biggest problems following my surgery was being able to de-stress. Eventually, I had to reduce all the external noises around me. I stopped watching television and listening to shows that were stressful, especially national network news. Instead, I began listening to downloaded inspirational books, searching through titles until I could find one with a positive message. I was so thankful that I could listen to these powerful messages, even if I was unable to read them because of my failing eyesight.

I was able to focus on avoiding negative distractions in order to be at peace with the world around me. I needed to block negative voices out of my life so that God's peace could dwell within me. I found that each time I listened and re-listened to these books, I found new lessons that have been so helpful in dealing with the stress of my situation.

Following my surgery, I found that I was extremely emotional, which in addition to the inner pain brought about by emotional responses, also hurt my body. I couldn't talk to family members because I was just too emotional. It hurt to cry.

John had to take over responsibilities that had been mine for over 50 years: preparing meals (most of which I couldn't eat anyhow), doing dishes, shopping, housekeeping, and just about everything else.

Eventually I was able to get to our living room using my walker. I would roll down the hall and sit, with John's help. As wonderful as John is in so many ways, he hasn't proven to be much of a cook, and all of this was as new for him as it was for me. I have clear memories of sitting on the couch waiting for John to make toast. After watching him burn three batches, I broke out in tears – this is how emotional I was. Finally, on the fourth try, John managed to make perfect toast. We laughed about it later, but not at the time.

By the time Christmas was getting close, we found we had waited too long to find a decent Christmas tree. A local nursery had one small evergreen left – one we could later plant and watch grow – and John brought it home. Although it was just a small, "Charlie Brown" tree, we found that by placing it on a round table and stringing lights from the very top all the way to the floor of our covered porch, we could light up the mountain night, displaying a much more impressive image than it probably deserved.

I was receiving mixed recommendations from my medical advisors. My surgeon and my oncologist both wanted me to undergo chemo and radiation therapy. My primary care physician, who totally "gets" MCS, said doing so would kill me. My surgeon said he had gotten "everything he could see or feel" but thought treatment would better my chances.

I decided to avoid putting massive doses of toxic chemicals into my body and place my fate in God's hands. Having better quality of life for a shorter period of time would, in my opinion, be better than having a longer, but much more miserable life.

Once I had retrained myself in life's basic functions, like walking unaided, I sought ways to increase my energy. Dr. B had mentored under a physician nearby who specialized in alternative treatments for chemical sensitivity. I signed up with him and made many trips to his office throughout the spring and summer of 2019. His staff gave me intravenous injections consisting of vitamin C and "magpacks."

I found this combination of ingredients to be very helpful in making me feel better, if not doing anything to address my cancer.

The summer of 2019 was the most amazing time in my memory. John and I, and Rowdy, had each other full time with no travel, no city council or other city distractions, no civic involvement of any kind. Just us, for the first time in more than a half a century of marriage.

Our days were spent walking on the beautiful mountain roads, swimming in our community lake, kayaking, and just enjoying the incredible home God had brought us to.

Then, in late September, I traveled to a nearby hospital on an early Sunday morning to have a PET scan, which had been ordered by my oncologist.

A few days later, I received a telephone call telling me my cancer was back.

I can't adequately describe what it is like hearing those words when I felt I still had so much left to do: Seeing another spring come to the mountains. Watching the plants and ground cover we had planted and nursed all summer come back to life. All the things we had talked about now turned to uncertainty.

What does this have to do with Multiple Chemical Sensitivity? I have no way of knowing whether the standard follow-up treatments to cancer would have given me more years, but I am confident that MCS prevented me from ever finding out. When your body reacts so violently to perfume, the last thing you want to do is introduce destructive chemicals that are so hard on people who don't even suffer from this condition.

We will never know.

I remember Thanksgiving 2019 – one year to the day since John and I walked out of the hospital and made our way home.

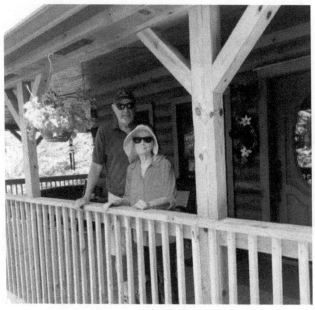

Fall of 2019, cancer had returned but Sandy and John had not yet shared the news with family.

I had known of my cancer's return for two months but had shared this with almost no one. Our next-door neighbor, a physician, and our neighbor across the lake, a Baptist minister, had both been supportive and we are blessed to have had them close.

As I reflected back on Thanksgiving a year ago and all that had happened since, I felt moved to write a positive, encouraging message to the people I loved. These are people I would soon be sharing a much more personal and difficult message with.

Gratitude at Thanksgiving

One year ago – Thanksgiving day 2018 – John and I were coming back from the hospital after my cancer surgery.

My hospital stay had been dismal, and we were leaving the hospital as soon as we could to get me into a chemical-free and fragrance-free environment – our new home on Melrose Mountain.

I was able to walk up the ramp to our new home with John's help. (We had moved into our home three weeks before we headed to the hospital.)

Prior to Monday morning's surgery, I thought I was ready to meet God in heaven.

The year since has been filled with many painful experiences.

But in spite of that pain, the past twelve months have been among the most wonderful and incredible years of our lives.

78

As we watch one year come to a close, and another, with so much unknown lying ahead of us, we are both filled with gratitude.

We have both slowed down our pace in spite of all that is going on in the world around us.

Following my surgery, I have experienced so much that I had not anticipated and now find that I appreciate little things that I had previously taken for granted.

Learning to walk again not using my walker and eventually able to pick things up off the floor.

Waking up each day with a sense of renewal and gratitude.

Feeling John's constant support and understanding.

And in the spring of this year, planting a variety of beautiful flower gardens and ground covers, and watching them spring up to cover the ground around our home.

The challenge of working together to be sure our 200 plus plants have enough water every day during the dry season.

The welcome sound of rain on our roof and watching our plants thrive as it poured down on them.

Sitting on our covered porch together, listening to the frogs jumping into the lake and loving the peaceful quiet living on the mountain.

Taking walks with our faithful companion Rowdy, the mountain cat, watching him bound up steep hillsides while we walk slowly on the road.

Talking to John about everything, knowing he was listening and supportive.

This is just a small list of things I am thankful for at this special time of year.

My book, when it is written will contain more about the special people that have shared in our life this year.

Most importantly, this year I've come to finally recognize the importance of Jesus Christ in our lives. I have been able to study God's Word and see how He has touched our lives in so many different ways.

I understand now that God had work to do on me before taking me to my forever home. He's still working on me. I am filled with gratitude for God giving me this extra time to bring Him more fully into our lives.

This year, as you make your list about the things you are thankful for, know that you are such an important part of ours.

—Sandy Major, 11/27/2019

I wanted to share this message with my children and their children, my brothers and sisters and all their families before I would have to tell them what I had not yet shared. My time with them, as my doctors had told me, would be measured in months and not years.

But I would be telling them. I was able to write handwritten letters to both our children. The essence of those letters was put into an email that was sent to other family members. So, everyone knew.

Here is the letter my family received:

Dear Family,

I'm writing to you because this is a difficult thing for me to talk about, even on the telephone. It is a sad subject, but for me it is also a peaceful one.

We learned recently that my cancer is back and there will not be any further alternative treatments. There is no way of knowing how soon the end is coming for me, but both John and I have accepted this and are at peace with it.

We are grateful for having shared so many wonderful years together. As I said in my Thanksgiving note, this last year has brought us closer together and closer to Jesus Christ than ever.

We have always looked at family as a precious gift, regardless of the miles and even years that have separated us. Watching each of your families grow over all these years has been a very special part of our lives.

I hope to look down from Heaven on each of your families as you continue to grow in your own special God-given gifts.

I tried to avoid sharing this news at such a happy time of year, but unfortunately I had to write now while my mind is clear.

John continues to help me, and I appreciate that he has respected my wishes throughout this time. We have also been in touch with our local Hospice and are in the process of looking into our long-term care insurance policy to see what help might be available there.

This past year has been an exceptionally happy one for me. Thanksgiving was a wonderful time for both John and me. We are also thankful for the incredible Christmas season that we are sharing together.

We are especially grateful that, for the first time in our lives, we are understanding the teachings of Jesus Christ and the meaning of His Grace.

I really want for you all to be happy for us and only wish for you to find God's Grace for yourself.

You may share this letter with other members of your family.

I will miss each of you, but I am looking forward to joining Jesus in my forever home when the time comes, whenever that may be.

I send this with love and in the name of our Lord Jesus Christ.

—Sandy

No one ever knows just how to react to news like this. Some wanted to catch the next plane while others just admitted that they really didn't know what to do.

But then it was Christmas again – our third since making the trip from Tybee. This year we had more than enough time to find a proper Christmas tree, although our little "Charlie Brown tree" from last year was doing just fine growing in his new home by our fence.

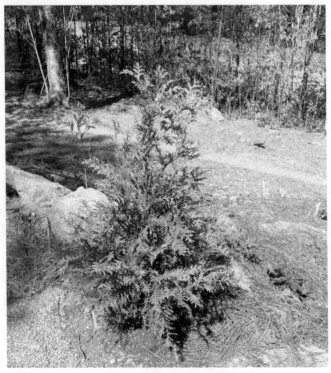

As was Sandy's wish, the little Charlie Brown tree has now been planted in a sunny spot with a view of the lake where it can bring shade and enjoyment for future generations.

John called around and found a local store that had just received their first batch of trees. I honestly thought that the one he brought home had been sent by God. It was perfect. He placed it in the same place on our porch where Charlie had been last year. Its lights, seen through our great room window, could be seen shining its message of hope and joy in the Savior we honor during this season.

One by one, I have been able to once again speak with my family. During the Christmas holidays, our daughter and her wonderful family visited us, as they had planned for months. I was able to spend time with both her and her husband, and with my grandchildren as well. Then, in early January, our son and his beautiful daughter spent time with us, and my sister has been here, helping out for weeks.

As February approaches, I guess it's time to finally take down the tree.

Maybe we can let the lights shine for just a few more nights.....

Note: Sandy passed away, in the home she loved, on February 8, 2020. This book is dedicated to her memory and to all those she hoped it could help in their struggles with this terrible affliction.
John Major

Chapter 15

REMEMBERING SANDY

In the preceding pages, Sandy told her story from her perspective – from that of a person who had gone from a dynamic, involved community and business leader to someone whose medical condition imposed almost complete withdrawal from everything and everyone that had previously filled her life.

It is important that the reader understand this illness, not only from that viewpoint, but also from that of those whose lives she impacted.

We have, therefore, included this final chapter, written after her death, in which some of the many people who knew and loved Sandy can describe how MCS had impacted them personally.

As her husband and the closest witness to this tragedy, I will go first:

* * *

"She's gone."

I remember choking on those words as I tried to let my daughter know that her mother had, finally, expectedly, passed away. I sat in our living room – in the beautiful log home we had built and loved over the last 16 months – where I had sat for most of the past several weeks, not sure of what I would do in the next 20 minutes or 20 years. I had sat in this same chair, watching the only person I had really known love with slowly, sometimes painfully, fade from me.

Just short of one week earlier, Sandy had positioned herself on our couch – the couch we had picked out together for our new home – and told me "I know what I have to do." From that time on, from Sunday afternoon until Saturday night, she didn't eat and drank only small amounts of water when she took pain medicines. That would come less and less frequently as the week progressed.

I guess she was ready to bring this terrible chapter in her wonderful life to its inevitable conclusion sooner rather than later. Our doctor-neighbor had looked in on her several times and explained that the end, for Sandy, was close. Without food and especially without adequate hydration, she would gradually slip into a sleep from which she would not wake.

Not by design, at least not by my design, our son was with me when Sandy died. Less than an hour earlier, he had gotten on his knees and prayed for God to take her, that she was ready. I guess God answered that prayer, even if He had passed on so many of my earlier ones. Having him close, and soon after, having my daughter and her family close, has made the unbearable bearable.

Hospice was amazing. Even though it was after 10:00 p.m. on a Saturday night three miles up a mountain road, the on-duty nurse said, in response to my call, "I'll be there within an hour." And she was.

She took care of whatever had to be done with Sandy. I'm not sure what all was involved, but within about an hour after she arrived, now approaching midnight, two men in suits from the local funeral home arrived and it was finally over.

Having helped Sandy put her MCS story in writing, since her sensitivity to light kept her from typing the words herself, I wanted to share the story from a different perspective. In the book Sandy says that it isn't just the sufferer who suffers. The impacts of this affliction stretch from the victim into the lives of everyone they love and who loves them.

She was always a fighter. Her biological father was shot down in WWII, leaving her mother five months pregnant with Sandy. When Sandy was five, her mother remarried to a wonderful man who gladly adopted Sandy and raised her as his own.

She was active in high school and entered Michigan State University as a freshman in 1962.

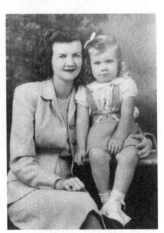

Sandy pictured with her widowed mother, Doris.

So did I.

A Saturday night mixer in my dorm brought us together in a random encounter. After asking her to dance and then dancing every song that came after, I walked her back to her dorm. By the time we got there, we knew we had something special. That was May 1963. I proposed four months later, and we married in June of 1964.

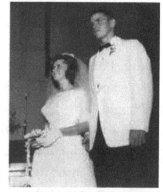

John and Sandy were married in June of 1964.

After graduating I went on active duty in the Navy. God blessed us with two wonderful children, both being born while I was in Vietnam.

Following my discharge from the Navy, my career took us to Pittsburgh, where our children were able to grow up in a stable and loving home, provided mostly by Sandy, since I was usually traveling somewhere with my job.

While I was flying around the country and around the world, Sandy was quietly but determinedly creating her own legacy that remains in place today. In the Pittsburgh area, she established a childcare center, and set it on a course that continues today.

After we discovered Deep Creek Lake in Maryland and purchased a home there, Sandy was hired by the local college as a small business counselor, helping aspiring entrepreneurs get started in their own busi-

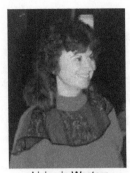

Living in Western Maryland, Sandy stayed busy with teaching, small business counseling, and civic activities while John traveled with his business.

ness or, in some cases, talking them out of it.

I watched in wonder as an idea for a small business incubator center, where new enterprises could share resources and enjoy cheap rent to help them get started, was born. The idea went from a grant proposal, which she wrote, to architectural plans to construction of a beautiful center attached to the local college.

When it opened, Sandy was the first director of the center.

In 1997, a small business counselor conference brought Sandy to Savannah, Georgia. From there she discovered Tybee Island, and another move started to take form. After I retired in 2000 and we started

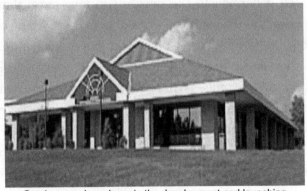

Sandy was a key player in the development and launching of a small business incubator center in Western Maryland.

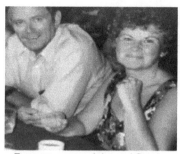

For many years, John and Sandy lived a magical life on Tybee Island, enjoying the beach community and participating in many local activities.

our own small business consulting company, we sold our Deep Creek property and moved to Tybee.

For 15 years, we lived a magical life on Tybee. We were both involved in local government and community activities, and I thought, again, that I was where I would be. Where we would be forever.

Then came the Lake Tahoe wedding, the Tiki Torch party, and two hurricanes with their toxic cleanups. By 2015, Sandy had developed full-blown Multiple Chemical Sensitivity. Going through all the suffering and humiliation that this crippling condition brings is a terrible thing to experience. To watch it happen to the person you love more than anything in the world, to be unable to do anything to help, to have to just sit there and watch this happen to this special person, is heartbreaking, every day, in every circumstance. Wherever you go, whatever you try to plan, whoever you invite into your home – every aspect of your life is defined by MCS.

One by one, Sandy dropped out of the activities that had been so important to her. Church was no longer an option. City committees and activities became impossible.

I remember the Thanksgiving just after our daughter and her family had moved into their new home. This one especially excited our daughter because it was the home she planned to retire in.

Sandy and I had made reservations to visit her new home and spend the holiday with our daughter and her family. As the date approached, she finally said to me "I don't think I can do it."

Thoughts of crowded airports, recirculating airplane air, rental cars that may or may not be tolerable, all were just too much for her to think about.

I called my daughter and said we would not be coming. Sandy never got to see the beautiful home.

Any trips we would take would involve calls ahead to multiple hotels to try and find one that would agree to our special cleaning requirements – non-toxic products, sheets, towels, and pillowcases washed in vinegar or borax, no fragrance sprays, on and on.

Many would just tell us they were not equipped to make these adjustments; others would agree and then not do it.

Imagine arriving in a hotel late at night after a long flight from somewhere, expecting, hoping to find a room that will not send you into a downward physical and emotional spiral, and finding that they just didn't get it.

What would you do?

91

Having people into our home was equally challenging. Friends and acquaintances generally weren't too big a problem – we just stopped seeing them. Family was another matter. We would talk, email, and text all our special requirements before their visit and it would usually work out satisfactorily, although some of the girls did have to take a lemon juice shampoo upon arrival to get the smell of their last treatment out of their hair.

Maintenance people would usually try, although if their previous call had been to the home of a heavy perfume user or smoker, they could be bringing some of that into our home. Sandy would retreat to the back bedroom where she would withdraw until they were finished. We would then open windows and doors and turn on fans until whatever lingering fragrances were gone. Not too bad in the warm temperatures, but rather brutal when it was cold.

After Tybee's two hurricanes and our move to Western North Carolina, we found ourselves in a new area where we knew no one and were unable to immerse ourselves in the local community. We tried church but each time were welcomed by well-meaning members with freshly applied perfume or cologne, always wanting to hug us into their fold. While Sandy was getting quite good at using her stiff-arm, and I was able to explain that "we don't hug," it proved too difficult and always with unfortunate consequences for her, for the rest of the day.

I wouldn't trade the two years we had, first building, then living in, our beautiful home in Western North Carolina for anything. Sandy described her joy in walking, kayaking, swimming and all the other things that we were able to do. Together. In almost 56 years of marriage, we had never had that kind of time or opportunity for it to be just us, and with time to do things we loved to do.

There was no place I would rather be. There was no one I would rather be with.

During this special time, the MCS wasn't so big a problem. We kept ourselves isolated from most of the world, on the top of a mountain, just us. Our family knew the rules and were a blessing when they visited us.

The bigger problem, the one that would be the final problem, was cancer.

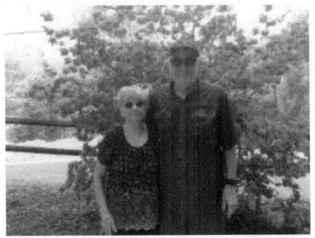

The natural beauty of Western North Carolina combined with the fresh mountain air, made moving there an easy decision.

We were planning to move into the new home in October 2018. She was diagnosed in September and scheduled for massive surgery in November.

The last days of 2018 were days of recovery and relearning for Sandy. I watched her go from a walker to a cane and then back to full capacity. As spring of 2019 approached, we did not give much thought to her cancer – the doctor said he had gotten everything he could "see or feel," and she seemed to be feeling pretty good.

We made full use of the facilities our community had to offer. She loved to walk down to the lake – directly across from our home – and swim or kayak. Sometimes I would swim with her; other times I would just sit on the dock and watch her smooth, strong strokes.

My conclusion from all of this is that if you are living with a person with MCS, it is possible to live a wonderful life. That is, provided you are willing to withdraw from just about everything society has to offer, and are fortunate enough to be able to have a home where you can escape all the invasive toxic products that put your life-partner over the edge.

Our life on the mountain was good. Then, in September 2019, Sandy's oncologist insisted that she have a PET scan to follow up on something he had seen in an earlier CAT scan.

A few days later, we got the call. The cancer was back.

She never tried to say that MCS caused the cancer. But it is clear to me, as it was to her, that MCS kept her from even trying to keep it at bay.

I was with her in her oncologist's office when he was telling her that she should try chemotherapy. Just smaller doses to start out.

I was with her when her primary physician told her that with her MCS, any amount of chemo would kill her.

Both agreed on one thing – without this treatment, which her doctor thought would be fatal – we were talking months, not years.

She wrote her Thanksgiving message to our immediate family and her siblings, then, as Christmas approached, she sent, rather had me send, her final message to everyone.

I was aching as I transcribed her words. She, on the other hand, was exhibiting strength and resolve that I could only look at in awe. Once Sandy had accepted her fate, she went about making sure that I had the basic skills I would need to exist on my own.

Then, just as I had watched her and helped her after her surgery as she practiced and learned to use her walker, then her cane, and finally, to walk unassisted as we went through each day together, I now saw her go from walking down our driveway to the lake to using her cane to get there, then her cane and my arm, and finally not being able to walk the roads at all. For as long as she could, she would walk around our yard, stopping wherever a bumblebee or especially a butterfly might be dining on the nectar of one of the many plants she had carefully placed around the yard.

Our children and grandchildren visited over the Christmas holidays. Sandy was only able to sit and talk with them in short intervals. Seeing them, seeing what wonderful adults our grandchildren were becoming brought her great joy and comfort.

But now, as I had told our daughter, she was gone.

The local funeral home created a guest book where friends and family could try to express how they felt in learning of Sandy's passing. One in particular captured her legacy. It's from a small Maryland business owner who Sandy had worked with, prayed with, and encouraged to use her God-given talents to open her own business. A business that continues to flourish today.

Dear John and Family,

I just got the paper and saw that Sandy passed. I am so sad to read about this. Sandy was one of the biggest influences in my life. She was an amazing mentor, friend, and teacher.

She always gave me a push to be a better employer and businessperson.

Sandy did so much for Garrett County and Garrett College and worked on so many committees like the

Job Fair, Cool Tools, GEIC, Deep Creek Lake Business Association and The Chamber of Commerce.

What a loss there is with Sandy gone.

Love, Garrett County, MD

This person captures the thoughts and feelings I have heard so many times since that night in February. With Sandy, life was never about making a lot of money. It was always, and only, about helping other people.

Fifty-six years ago, God gave me an angel. On February 8, 2020, He took her back.

It's not just the sufferer of MCS who suffers. It's every member of that person's family, the grandkids who don't understand why grandma can't be at their graduation. It's the children who are so eager to share their new home with you and can't really understand why you can't come.

It's all the organizations that would have benefited so much from your contributions that were never made because you were not able to be there.

It is especially the person or persons who love you the most and find themselves having to withdraw from a world they thought they would have been living in to provide the physical and emotional support you will need as you face this terrible condition.

In her final months and weeks, Sandy was focused on getting her story written. Sharing in her efforts was a painful but wonderful experience as she would dictate to me, then read and edit my attempts at capturing her thoughts and, finally, my seeing the acceptance in her eyes.

Now, as I try to capture my own raw feelings, I can only pray that her purpose in writing the book can be realized. It was her hope that someone will read her words and understand that MCS is real, and take action to make sure they, and those they love, will never have to endure what she did.

—John Major

* * *

It's useful to look at MCS and its impact on a family through the eyes of the children of the person with the condition. Our daughter Lisa was always family oriented, and spending time with those she loved was an important part of her life and still is.

Here are some of Lisa's memories.

For as long as I can remember, I've wanted to have a large family. I have so many wonderful memories of visiting my grandparents' house and spending time with my aunts and uncles – some of them weren't much older than me. My dad, mom, brother, and I would pack into our car, make the five-hour trip, and spend days at their house. My mom had five younger siblings, each of whom are now long since married and have children of their own. Many of these family members were also there, and I so enjoyed the carefree family gatherings: playing games, swimming in the pool, gathering around the fireplace, telling stories, grilling, eating together. These get-togethers were an impactful part of my upbringing and formed a big part of what became the important core of what I valued in life. As the years went by, these gatherings transitioned to either my parents' house or one of my aunts' houses, or we would all rent a vacation home together. So many people all together, so many good times, and so many memories. It seems like Mom was always the main organizer of these gatherings and kept herself in the middle of all of the activity.

I am positive that these gatherings influenced me to have a big family of my own and to continue these traditions. For many years, as an adult, my husband and I continued to participate in these family events, staying with my parents and eventually passing these important traditions on to our own children. However, over time, as the unrelenting nature of my mother's chemical sensitivity disorder progressed, getting together began to take on a whole new level of complexity. Even though we all did what we could to accommodate her limitations, looking back at this now, I realize how this insidious and unrelenting condition slowly took more and more of what I loved about my mom away from me, and away from my family. It makes me sad for all of us, and I can only imagine how hard it must have been from her perspective, to be robbed of so many things that she held dear.

Having a family member, especially a mom/ grandmother with multiple chemical sensitivity

99

disorder, impacts every member of the family. Simple things that are usually taken for granted turn into involved, complex events, if they can even happen at all. Planning a visit to my parents' house meant taking an inventory and making sure that all six members of our family and my son's fiancé had the proper scent-free shampoo, deodorant, soap, and other personal products. Several months before visiting, we would all make sure that we were washing our clothes in Free and Clear laundry detergent to get rid of any residual scents. Although my husband and I and two youngest children used this product anyway, the three oldest, living away from home on college budgets, usually used on a daily basis what was most affordable, which usually meant scented.

Several days before we would leave to visit them, we would begin using the fragrance-free personal products. We would also have to re-train ourselves not to use lotion, perfume, hairspray, or any other product that was typically a part of our everyday life. This may seem like a simple task; however, it is so easy to slip when it is something that you are used to doing every day, such as putting on hand lotion. Despite all of this preparation, purchasing the scent-free products to take with us and leaving the scented products at home, it was so easy to forget and make a mistake, such as using the soap or hand sanitizer in the public restroom during stops en route to their house. This simple error would then basically "undo" all of our previous efforts, as we would not be able to get near my mom as a result. If you could not pass her "sniff test," essentially, if she was able to smell any scent at all on you, you would have to keep your distance from her.

Sometimes, despite all of the planning and effort that we made, scents still remained. I remember an instance when we were visiting, and for some unknown reason, my son and his fiancé were never able to pass her test and therefore were not able to get near her. It's sad when everyone else was able to be close to my mom, they had to keep their distance. Although they understood this, on some level, I am sure emotionally it probably felt like some level of rejection. As frustrating as it was for all of us, I can't even imagine what it did to her.

When we bought our beautiful new home four years ago, I could not wait to have my parents visit. We talked in length about the measures I would take to remove scents from our home, such as cleaning with vinegar and water in preparation, removing all air fresheners, candles, etc., and making sure that all of their bedding and towels were washed in Free and Clear detergent. This visit never came about. The logistics of arranging everything, between the nine+ hour trip or even thinking of flying and staying at our house became more than my mom thought that she could handle. One bad interaction in a rest stop along the way, or sitting in toxic air in an airport, airplane or rental car, and the visit would be negatively impacted. With my mom not able to come, my dad was not able to either, since he had to stay back to assist her. It was hard watching the parents of my neighbors come into town and spend time with their grandkids knowing that my parents could not do the same.

Fortunately, we could still visit them, and we had a wonderful stay with them over the Christmas holiday of 2018, and again in the spring of 2019. We were looking forward to spending a good portion of the upcoming 2019 Christmas break with them when we got the devastating news that my mom was given a prognosis of only months to live. I remember, when we did get to visit with her, sitting there talking to her from a distance across her family room, it all felt so surreal, trying to take it all in, not knowing if this would be the last time I would see her (which it was), listening to her talk. I couldn't get too close physically, I couldn't hug her, even though I had prepared in every way that I could to remove all scents, we couldn't take a chance of making her any more uncomfortable. My husband and I and each of our kids got to spend limited time, each from a distance, with her during this visit as she could only handle so much interaction due to her discomfort and low endurance.

The mom that I grew up with had always been a vibrant, independent woman, who was always on the go. Watching her gradually lose her strength and withdraw from all the things she loved to do, including being with our family, was one of the hardest things I ever witnessed. I loved my mom. I miss her. What I do believe, however, is that time will soften my memories of the difficult challenges of these past five years, and that the core of who she was will be what I remember. The love, the laughter, the get-togethers, and all she did to make me the person I am will be how I will see and remember her.

* * *

Our son Rob had a special bond with Sandy, and here he shares some his favorite things about her and special memories.

Loving, caring, supportive, balanced, brave, strong and independent...these are some of the words that describe my mom.

It seems like she left her mark wherever she went. When I was growing up, her concern for others led her to starting and expanding businesses, creating educational platforms, and building incubation facilities for small businesses. She achieved these successes in environments where many times the odds were stacked against her.

While she was an amazing example of a career-minded woman, she always took the time for her family. My dad travelled most of the time for business that so much of the child raising responsibilities fell on her. I am sure that this was challenging at times, as I was a little ornery as a kid. But no matter what situation I got into, she was always there to help and support me. She had my back when I needed her help and advice in handling tough business and personal challenges as an adult.

I think her independence must have taken root when my dad was away serving our country in Vietnam up to a year at a time. She delivered both my sister and me while he was away. But when dad was back home I have so many fond memories of her orchestrating family activities, like picnics, fun dinners including fondue and fire pit grilling, card games, and relaxing vacations at Myrtle Beach. She was also there to support us with our cross-country and track meets, and band activities, always cheering us on.

The last several years of her life were tough on all of us, especially her. She was unable to travel to visit us, my sister or other family due to her illness. Even so, she kept a positive outlook, and she and dad always gave us an open invitation to visit them at their homes in Tybee Island, GA, and Tryon, NC, which was really special, as long as we came to town "fragrance free." At first, I found this a little odd, but after some time got used to the idea. I can remember her saying, "think about it Rob, why would you want to put toxic chemicals right against your body all day and night?" It sunk in, and we still wash in fragrance-free detergent today.

She must have known that she was near the end of her life here on earth, because she had my dad call me and request that I fly down to NC to pick up the Subaru Outback that she and dad had gifted to my daughter. In doing so, I was there with my dad during her last hours. One of the most special moments of my life was kneeling down beside her that last night, praying with her and assuring her that Jesus was ready for her to come home. Dad and I are convinced she planned it to happen this way.

Yes, my mom was a great planner. She made sure to teach dad how to operate all of the household appliances so that he could live comfortably, cooking and cleaning for himself after she was gone.

She always put others first, especially the ones she loved. After she passed, we learned that she had even tried to plan her own final arrangements with the funeral home. This was so typical of her. She was trying to make the difficult process as easy as possible for my dad.

I am so blessed to have Sandy Major as my mom. For her entire life, she was there supporting me no matter what, never judging or questioning.

I will miss her every day.

* * *

Sandy's sister Laura and brother-in-law Joe, who live in Lake Orion, Michigan, were able to be with us during her final days, and were more help to me than I can express. Joe read through the drafts of her book and offered valuable insight. I asked him to add his own memories of Sandy.

I am Joe, Sandy's brother-in-law. I married her younger sister, Laura, born 11 years after Sandy. I have always

105

and only known Sandy as "Sandy and John". I rarely used or even spoke her last name.

Before I married Laura, we visited Sandy and John at their home in Gibsonia, Pennsylvania. Laura was excited to have me meet her "big" sister [said the 5-foot-3 girl about her 5-foot-1 sibling], and I suspect be approved or disapproved. The visit was wonderful, as the home had a small mineral spring creek running through the house, which fascinated me. They had two very big St. Bernard dogs, several horses, and a large, wooded lot. They also had two beautiful energetic children. It was instantly clear that the ringmaster of the circus was Sandy.

Sandy had a soft yet firm, if not insistent, tone of voice. She was at once a great listener and a good reader of people, as all great mothers need to be. Her eyes truly twinkled when she laughed, a genuine but modest laugh. I must have passed the audition, as Laura and I did marry.

My knowledge of Multiple Chemical Sensitivity began with my introduction to it via Laura's sister-in-law, Linda. She had become sensitive to things, such as colognes, deodorants, and other scented products leading to disabling migraines.

I did not become aware of Sandy's fight with MCS until she became a hurricane refugee. Sandy and John lived happily (and busily) on Tybee Island, near Savannah, Georgia, for many years with no issues other than Sandy managing John's diabetes and diet. She did this well, like a drill sergeant, but with a soothing voice. After the hurricane clean up began, Laura told me Sandy was now reporting the same problems as Linda. When Laura and I visited them in Tybee that year, I was introduced to unscented soaps and shampoos, as well as laundry detergent (and no dryer sheets at all).

At first, it did not seem like a big issue for me or for Sandy and John. Then the next hurricane came and with it the next clean-up campaign. Soon after, it was reported that Sandy and John had to escape their own home, as almost every chemical smell was triggering a reaction in Sandy. Being forced out of your own home due to a poorly understood illness seemed severe and unfair to me, but perhaps it was only temporary. Not so. It continued, and Sandy and John tried to find a new chemical-free ecosphere to live in. They sold their homes on Tybee in a rushed exit, leaving their friends behind.

They found significant relief in the foothills of North Carolina. Fresh air and very little development. By this time, Sandy and John had been touched by the cancer that would take Sandy. I was blessed to visit them one more time as her light was slowly but surely being extinguished.

I had to make sure that my clothes were washed in the right detergent. I did not take a shower for a couple of days, and had prepared by using "safe" shampoo and soap. I shaved with unscented hair conditioner.

It worked fine. The amount of preparation worked, as I did not trigger Sandy when I came to visit her on many occasions over the last few weeks that she was with us. I was also able to see all the special products that had to be used and extra precautions taken just to live a routine day. Even still, on occasion, it was not enough.

One of the first visiting nurses to see Sandy while the cancer began its final assault had to be turned away from her mission of mercy. Sandy's reaction was immediate. A fragrance warning was not heeded and, not trusting the process, Sandy refused additional help when Sandy and John most needed it. Another example of an innocent chemical intrusion was the cleaning person who had learned about the MCS situation that had invaded Sandy and John, and passed inspection previously. Unexpectedly, Sandy reacted to her one day. The cause was nail polish her niece had applied to her toes the day before. Sadly, Sandy was as sensitive as a bloodhound to certain scents that are an integral part of the chemistry of our everyday world. Unlike the hound, she could not turn it off and each new exposure brought on a miserable reaction. Putting myself in Sandy's shoes, or nose, would probably be like sticking my nose into the tailpipe of a running diesel engine bus.

My observation was that this seemingly "benign" condition is anything but. It alters a normal life in ways that are difficult to cope with. Knowing whether

her cancer was caused by the MCS, vice versa, or they were independent of each other would not have made life easier for Sandy and John. Sandy, however, seemed to fight the MCS as hard as she could, while accepting her cancer diagnosis with grace. I will always be curious to know which one was really more painful.

* * *

Laura, Joe's wife and Sandy's sister, reacted to a draft of my "memories" in a message that, while not intended for inclusion in the book, expressed her own feelings in a way that needed to be shared:

John, your addition to Sandy's book represents how strongly we all feel in our loss.

You talked about Sandy and swimming with her strong strokes. She was a great swimmer and loved being in the water. I remember watching her from the dock on Deep Creek Lake. After swimming she would lay flat on her back, floating while gazing up at the sky. Sandy appeared content and peaceful with just being in that moment.

Her strength, both physical and mental, was always evident – you just knew she was going to overcome any obstacle that arose, using all the "tools in her toolbox." She fought back, she took action, no matter what the issue was. She cared about and fought for, not only her own personal issues, but for the good of her family, friends, and communities. Whenever I come across a "little rubber ducky" in a store, I chuckle.

She just threw herself into causes that would make a positive change. Often, she was the initiator of that cause, the first to recognize the need, and persistently follow through to the end. Just one of the many things I admired about her – especially in contrast to how I handle things. We both care deeply, but she had that drive and persistence to initiate and follow through, pulling others along with her. I recognized early on that my sister was a leader, but also that she was wise, intelligent, and able to perceive needs that often went unrecognized by the rest of us.

One of the hardest things for me to witness was how her physical strength dwindled. How hard it must have been for you, John, to watch that happen. I only saw her toward the end, when physical strength was already taken from her. When I first saw her bundled up in sweaters, layers of socks, thick slippers, and even mittens under multiple blankets, I was shocked.

When I would hear her shuffle so very slowly down the hall past my bedroom at night, my heart broke into a million pieces. The sister that walked so confidently toward life was now reduced to this debilitating state. Yet in this suffering she still had her will, and faith in God to keep her going through the last journey.

How could she be so strong in this time of weakness with the pain that wracked her body? Steadfast in her faith when I, her siblings, and father would question God's plan. My older sister was still teaching me how to live, and by her example, how to die.

* * *

110

Sandy had five siblings. We named our daughter after Lisa, the youngest girl in the family who was the flower girl in our wedding and grew up with our children more like a cousin than an aunt. Lisa and her husband, Carlos, had visited us in North Carolina, fell in love with the area, and purchased a home in a nearby town. I am sure they were thinking we would all enjoy a long retirement together. The following are just some of Lisa's memories of Sandy.

> I always looked up to Sandy. She was the oldest daughter, and I was the youngest. I remember spending summers with her and her family, and I will forever cherish those memories. Sandy always made things fun and interesting at family gatherings. We had great family reunions at every home she and John owned.
>
> When Sandy first contracted MCS, she did her best to adjust, but over time I could see how it robbed her of many things, including her family. At first it was difficult for her to be around us all, and eventually it came down to our individual families just being able to visit her in small numbers.
>
> There was the list that was always sent to us from John or Sandy before every visit about what to avoid using – fragrant shampoo, laundry detergent, etc. Although we tried very hard, it seemed she would always detect something on us. We learned that just because a product label says "non-fragrant," it does not necessarily mean there is no fragrance, especially

to someone who is as sensitive as Sandy was.

The last year and a half, my husband and I were fortunate to spend more time with the Majors because, like them, we had fallen in love with North Carolina. We had spent many long weekends looking for our own retirement home, even though we have a few more years to work. I cherished my time with Sandy, yet I always missed the physical touch she could not bear. I missed hugging her hello and goodbye. You never realize how important human touch is until you do not have it.

We ended up buying a home 45 minutes away from the Majors, and we were hopeful that Sandy would live through her cancer ordeal, so we could spend time in our retirement with them. Tragically, that did not happen.

The last time I saw Sandy was in early January 2020. I had to always sit about 8 feet away and I was only able to spend about 15 minutes with her for each of my three visits during that week. Her total focus during those visits was on this book. She was driven to finish it before she died.

I remember the day I drove to Michigan to tell our father that Sandy's cancer had returned. Sandy and Dad had not been able to see each other because of her MCS and his age, 95. He mentioned that he had a dream a few days before about seeing Sandy and holding her. He just wished he could hold her one more time.

Human touch and closeness – we all need it. Even

though it had been a few years since Sandy hugged me, she gave me a great gift in October 2019. As we were saying goodbye after one of our visits, she hugged me goodbye. The cancer had returned, and she knew it, but wouldn't share it with us for another two months. I am forever grateful for that hug, and for my sister Sandy.

* * *

The last time Sandy was able to get together with her brothers and sisters for their father's 90th birthday. She was unable to be there for Dale's 95th.

Kathy is Sandy's sister and is second in line of the siblings. Here she shares some memories.

Sandy, now our Angel... was my big sister with whom I shared a room and a bed until she became a ninth grader. We were extremely different yet very close at the same time. Mom had gotten a picture for our room; it was of two southern girls, one brunette and one blonde in beautiful southern fashion, and it brought up a fun rivalry between Sandy (a blond) and me (a brunette). We constantly joked as to which girl in the picture was smarter, better looking, etc. Ironically, we both ended up living in the south.

I tried to live up to Sandy's example, but she was darn near perfect. Always calm and the voice of reason. She was an avid reader and had great grades, while the rest of the Brown family struggled a bit in school. More than once Dad said, "I wish you could be more like your sister (in school grades)." Sandy was just more gifted and motivated, so we went on our merry pathways in life, always loving and respecting each other. Frequently, I bounced ideas off her for advice, knowing she would have my best interest at heart.

We have always been a family of huggers – large family, large happy hugs at all our get-togethers and small occasions. It ceased when MCS took over – we were doing social distancing before it became a necessary trend in 2020. Considering all the side effects MCS caused Sandy personally, not being able to hug or even touch her was a major change for me,

114

yet small in comparison to her problems. Bravely she would go out to lunch with us on our visits, and she'd try to avoid perfume smells and wear big floppy hats and dark sunglasses to keep the light from her eyes because of her cataracts. Not too much later, she and John had to up and leave their home for a remote wooded area. We›ve missed their presence here in the Coastal Empire immensely.

The news that she had uterine cancer hit really hard. We all wanted to save her, but the follow-up chemo was deemed too dangerous because of the MCS. Ultimately the cancer claimed her with a huge assist from MCS.

She was my big sister, a teacher, a businesswoman and a volunteer – always there, always dependable, calm, and creative, and her passing leaves a big hole in my heart and many others.

I am a gardener and whenever I see a yellow butterfly, of which there are many, I think fondly of Sandy and her happy angel spirit, no longer bothered with pain and earthly matters.

* * *

Linda, wife of Sandy's brother David, is a long-term MCS sufferer and had these final thoughts.

Sandy is a hero. She spent her last weeks on this earth cancer-ridden but without pain medication, in order to get this book written. Her intention was to support, assist, and guide sufferers with this illness, and to help non-sufferers understand it.

True to Sandy's nature she made valuable contributions to other people's lives right up until her passing; and through her efforts in writing this book, she will continue to touch many people's lives for years to come.

Appendix A
Illness Differences, Spreading, Progression, and Coping Tips: More from Linda B.

You have read Sandy's words, heard part of her story, and discovered how life was going well for her and then Multiple Chemical Sensitivity hit. She spoke of the illness as having a five-year duration, how distressing it was, that she suspected its cause to be from long-term toxic exposure, how it manifested, and the devastating cost in terms of her cancer and premature death. You also read of my experience with the illness, and may have noticed the similarities and differences between our experiences. I believe that it was primarily the chemicals and other petroleum products within perfume that caused my MCS, and my duration of the illness has been 30 years to date. You will see later in this section, that many of the ingredients found in perfume and other fragranced products have recently been found to be very toxic, and that some non-profits are involved in trying to change laws which should lead to improvement in the fragrance industry. (Details of other toxic chemicals are found in further appendixes, and you are encouraged to reduce your toxic load from any source.)

You will also find reference to a research document in this section which involved analysis and diagnostic evidence of MCS sufferers (as well as a control group), and reference to the study's defined stages of MCS symptoms. Both Sandy and I were in the final "Deterioration" stage which gives credence to MCS contributing

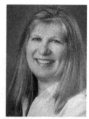

Linda Brown, Sandy's sister-in-law and long-time MCS sufferer.

to or causing our cancer and lung disease. This information is not documented to scare you. Sandy and I totally empathize with you.

Our hope is to inform, give you facts and tools that we did not have, and help you see that you should take the illness seriously (and to also help those who wish to understand and/or accommodate you). You will find that many doctors do not know enough about this syndrome – it needs more research, then findings would need to be detailed and disseminated into the medical community. I believe we have documented the seriousness of the syndrome and, hopefully, inspired you to be your own best advocate.

Some Differences and Spreading of Reactions

I further would like to discuss the differences between Sandy and others I knew with MCS. All shared sensitivity to perfumes, but there were differences with our sensitivities to various products, whether toxic or not.

I once thought if I could handle a product anyone could – not so. Sandy once suggested a body soap that she used; however, I could not tolerate the scent on myself nor others in my household using it. My sensitive hairdresser who was less sensitive than me, could not tolerate a shampoo I was using. That was surprising to me, because other than an initial mild scent while I was shampooing, I could not smell it; and neither could my husband (who I often ask for opinions because my sense of fragrances has changed through the years). Sometimes I could only smell a chemical rather than the scent the product was intended to present. This was not my first experience with someone reacting to a product I was using. The other time involved a man who would sneeze (the same reaction my hairdresser exhibited) with another shampoo I used. In the second example, the product was a natural-citrus scented shampoo, which I found easier to tolerate than flowery or heavy musk-like smells. Both instances were lessons for me (and I am thankful there are now very good unscented shampoos on the market.)

First lesson, if I am asking others to refrain from using scents, I clearly do not want to be emitting any detectable scent (whether or not the scent seems to be mild by my standards). Second, other MCS "sensitives" can and do have different triggers than mine. Third, why do I react strongly to not only the chemicals in perfumes but also to flowers? When I was exposed to fragrant fresh flowers, I had MCS-type reactions to them, which had not been the case when I was a child or young adult.

Before I go into this third item, I want to mention the triggers that other "sensitives" had disclosed to me. My dental hygienist with MCS could not go into a tire store (OK – petroleum related), nor could she handle the smell of a bakery (huh?). Sandy could not pump her own gasoline (not a big surprise), but she also could not tolerate the smell of chlorine from a swimming pool (a chemical not related to petroleum). Obviously, my problems with some plastics fit the petroleum category, but my problems with flowers do not. What I have learned is that "this type of cross-reaction or sensitivity to unrelated materials is called generalization or spreading" in MCS; and it is a "well-documented phenomenon. In true allergy, whereby a person with an allergy to one material can become truly allergic to another material which may or may not be related."[1] It is further explained that our immune system antibodies recognize a part or

---

1 Excerpt and paraphrase found on the site https://multiplechemicalsensitivity.org HOW REAL IS MCS article

a feature of an antigen (irritant) molecule, and if another molecule contains a matching feature it will attach to our antibodies binding site and produce an allergic reaction.

My reactions to flowers were akin to my MCS symptoms (not typical to my allergy symptoms), and I suggest you avoid any non-chemical products that produce MCS symptoms in you, just as you would fragrance or other chemicals you are sensitive to. Trust yourself and your instincts. I learned to understand my sensitivities and reactions, and now virtually all of them are publicly documented as causes or symptoms of MCS.

Other often-mentioned products that cause MCS symptoms include formaldehyde, carpet glue, and electricity; and MCS symptoms can include light sensitivity and food intolerances.

Progression of the Illness

For those of you who know or suspect that you have MCS, it is highly likely that your symptoms will progress, and the products that cause your symptoms (or the ability to detect them) will also likely increase. The good news is that the illness is becoming better known, that the number of good natural and unscented products is growing, and that you are taking the time to learn of MCS and learn what you can do to support yourself. First, I will detail how toxic fragrances are, then how serious the MCS illness is and how it can progress, then I will share some tips that I have learned from the trenches. Also, although I have no regrets, I may have done some things differently in the past had I known then what I know now, and I will share those thoughts with you.

A September 26, 2018, article titled "New Data Reveals One-Third of All Fragrance Chemicals Linked to Human, Environmental Harm" on the Women's Voices for the Earth website (www.womenvoices.org) states that "a third of all fragrance chemicals currently in use are either known to be toxic or considered potentially toxic." The article further stated that the BCPP (Breast Cancer Prevention Partners) disclosed "results of chemical testing of 140 popular U.S. personal care and cleaning products, revealed hundreds of toxic chemicals in the products, the majority of which were associated with the fragrance in the product." It went on to say that "three out of four of the toxic chemicals in the beauty and personal care products we tested were fragrance chemicals, and most of these toxic chemicals were not found on the product label."

I reviewed an article in the *Journal of Occupational and Environmental Medicine* website, titled "Multiple Chemical Sensitivity: Review of the State of the Art in Epidemiology, Diagnosis, and Future Perspectives[2], February 2018, by Rossi, S., and Pitidis, A. The

2 https://journals.lww.com/joem/Fulltext/2018/02000/ Multiple_Chemical_Sensitivity__Review_of_the_State.5.aspx

authors defined symptom stages of MCS and anyone who suffers from the syndrome would be considered within three stages that progress from sensitization to inflammation to deterioration. These three stages of chemical sensitivity could also be thought of as irritation, to illness, to damage.

Whether your symptoms came about from fragrances or another environmental contaminant is really of no consequence. Perhaps some of the tips mentioned below will help you to slow or to avoid entering the next stage.

Prior to moving forward, I will tell you of my progression through the stages to provide an example of how it could happen, and perhaps answer some questions the symptom stages could generate. I did not understand what was making me sick, so I did not avoid fragrances until my (suspected) eighth year of symptoms. At year four, I was substantially ill, and had been diagnosed with chronic fatigue and immune dysfunction syndrome (CFIDS). I believe I was having symptoms that "oscillated for days, if not weeks," and which is mentioned in stage 2 of the study document. In year nine, I began allergy shots that would definitely put me in stage 2. In year 25, I was diagnosed with very mild COPD caused by emphysema, which in year 29 had progressed to moderate COPD lung disease, which would definitely put me in stage 3. I had recognized in those last four to five years that I was getting short of breath (asthma) after an exposure, or that I sometimes had substantial lung congestion after a longer or stronger exposure, but I did not understand that I had asthma, and did not suspect that my COPD could worsen, because I was told my "mild COPD" would not be an issue within my expected lifetime. I believe this is an example of how misunderstood MCS has been and that it is not taken seriously in the medical field. It also shows how quickly symptoms can worsen if sensitive people do not avoid their triggers as much as is possible.

Coping Tips

MCS is a serious illness which will greatly impact people who are afflicted with it and possibly affect friends, family, coworkers, and others around them. These tips are primarily meant for the afflicted.

First of all, you will need to grieve. Give yourself permission. There is a loss of your health as you knew it, and in your capability to navigate your current world, and a certain fear of the unknown (what will your future be like?). Not only is this a whole lot to accept, but your emotions may be intensified occasionally by exposures causing feelings of sadness, anger, or hopelessness. Realize there are stages to grieving, and it is fine if you occasionally need to curl up or vent. Yet, those who are afflicted must carry on and do the best they can within their circumstances. Use what tools you can, and let others support you.

I believe that once you know you are sensitive to perfumed products, you should remove all of them from your environment as soon as possible. This would include all hand soaps, dishwasher soaps, cleansing agents and, most of all, laundry products. I recommended specific personal and laundry products earlier, and can recommend a plant-based, all-purpose cleaner called Puracy natural surface cleaner with green tea and lime, if you have no issues with either of those scents. Also, Seventh Generation, Open Nature, and Full Circle Market make good dishwashing products. Be aware that you may be accustomed to a product that you have used for a long time, and it may not seem offensive to you but could be affecting you, nonetheless. Do clean up your immediate environment ASAP by disposing of those products, or giving them away if you do not feel right about throwing them out.

Those closest to you may be able to wear perfume, a scented deodorant, or use a scented lotion when you are not around (even if you do not recommend it), but they will need to make sure their clothes (or seatbelt straps) have not absorbed the product's smell if they are to wear those clothes when you are nearby or if they ask to drive you somewhere. However, it is very probable that they will not be able to use scented laundry products if they want to stay in close physical contact with you, because those scents do not wash out. Scented laundry products leave odors on your clothes, in your washer and dryer, on your upholstery, even your hard chair surfaces, your house and car, and things you handle will smell strongly of them. Think of laundry products as staining or perfuming every fiber and crevice of those surfaces, and permeating your skin.

Instructions for removing laundered scents from clothes:

- Soak, then wash clothes in very hot water with unscented dish soap (you are trying to remove the scented oil from the material), and you may need to repeat the process.
- If the scent still lingers, bake the clothes in the sun, turn clothes, and repeat if necessary.

This works well with newly purchased clothes also.

It can be very difficult for those who are trying to understand and support you by not using offending products. They may have tried to accommodate you, and they do not know what they could have done differently. It's also possible they did forget something. It was sometimes helpful that my husband could "track down a scent," which would not have been possible for me. One thing to be very aware of is "transference." If you sit in a public chair, your clothes will pick up the scent of the clothes of others who previously sat in it. One of Sandy's sisters came to stay with us, and she had been using only unscented laundry products for years, yet I was reacting to a laundry product smell in her presence. We determined it was her suitcase that was transferring a scent to her clothes. She then

126

washed all of her clothes in our home, and we were fine. I do not have a keen sense of smell, but I have often thought if others could smell fragrance in a quantity of one part per million, I must be able to smell it in one part per billion. And that might not be far from the truth. The same article in the *Journal of Occupational and Environmental Medicine* article states that MCS "is a complex disease, a multisystem disorder that manifests as a result of exposure to various environmental contaminants (solvents, hydrocarbons, organophosphates, heavy metals) at concentrations below the 'Threshold Limit Value' (TLV) that are considered toxic doses for the general population." It would be hard for the unafflicted to understand our sensitivity towards something they cannot smell, or does not bother them, which might lead them to think that we are over-reacting.

It is ultimately the sensitive person's responsibility to help others understand what they can do to assist them. Perhaps it is too much to ask of some friends but, hopefully, you have family members who are willing to comply with your wishes. You could suggest they read an article posted on the Invisible Disabilities Association website, which explains how toxic perfume is and how it can affect those who are sensitive. It can be found at: https://invisibledisabilities.org/publications/chemicalsensitivities/whygofragrancefree/

You might also consider having an option of scent-free clothes stored at your home that friends/family members could change into. If need be, visits might only be possible when weather permits windows to be open, or out in the open air with the sensitive person upwind.

The ones trying to accommodate might understand the MCS sufferer better if they know that it is impossible for the sensitive to "forget" there's a triggering scent in their vicinity, because the scent overwhelms their senses. I became nervous around all scents, but found that if I was able to forget about a scent within minutes, it was non-toxic for me; however, if I could not get the scent out of my mind, it was an irritant for me and would generate symptoms.

The workplace can be bothersome. Your employers may not be very accommodating. They may try, but you may have coworkers who will not cooperate. Most of us need to work. You can try filters, masks, buying a product for a coworker to replace the hand lotion that is bothersome and appealing to them to try it, education, opening windows, sealing off a vent, asking to change offices or partners, changing jobs, retiring on disability, lawsuit, etc. Working in an office building was a struggle for me, even though I know many people tried to accommodate me. It only takes one person in your work area to spoil the clean air. It is helpful that the Environmental Protection Agency (EPA) and the Americans with Disabilities Act (ADA) recognize MCS. Good luck!

We discussed the difference between allergies and chemical sensitivity earlier. Even though allergy shots are not available or feasible for chemical sensitivities, I believe the 20 years I had gotten allergy shots (for foods, pollens, dust, and molds) were helpful, because they took some of the load off of my immune system. In my case, chemical sensitivity seemed to trigger immune reactivity to allergens, or perhaps it was an immune system malfunction that caused the allergies. Nevertheless, I believed the shots made me feel better, and my allergies reduced in severity because of them.

It may be worth noting that some people believe that food allergies exacerbate environmental sensitivities. As for me, I found it very helpful to avoid eating onions and garlic so that I could smell offending agents before I started reacting to them, and then to move from the area if possible. If you know of a food sensitivity, or just want to improve your diet, it might be worth a try to eliminate some foods and add others.

I know both Sandy and I were taking Zyrtec for many, many years. It would reduce the sinus congestion, ear pain, coughing, and migraines in my case often caused by exposures. As for migraines, they are their own monster, and would often affect and exhaust me for days. I found Triptans to be a godsend in reducing the pain and side effects. If your doctor recommends and prescribes them, I suggest giving them a try (I would get relief with a half-dose within hours).

Whenever going out in public, it may be helpful to wear a scarf around your neck to place over your nose and mouth when encountering an offending scent. Of course, face masks are much more common to wear since the COVID-19 outbreak.

I am fortunate that I am not hypersensitive to carpets as Sandy was, but do be aware of fragranced carpet pads and commercial carpet cleaning products. You may decide to avoid any chemicals that you can, but if you will be remodeling, take extra precautions to learn of the new products. If you do a quick search for Naphtha, a toxic hydrocarbon, you may be shocked to find how many personal care and household products have it as an ingredient. The appendixes to this book include the Top Five Toxic Chemicals. You can find other ways you can live a cleaner life in the appendix What Can I do? Fortunately, much information is available for MCS sufferers, and some sources are listed in the Helpful Resources appendix.

I once read something like "when you are in darkness, it can be hard to see the light." I am sure you will do what you can to navigate this illness, but also recognize and be grateful for what you do have. Take time to focus on the light. This is your life, and since the human condition is to have challenges as well as blessings, you will get through it. Know that you are not alone. Sandy and I wish you the very best.

Appendix B
HELPFUL RESOURCES

In preparing this book, and as I searched the internet and literature over the past several years, many of these sources provided valuable information for me. I am listing as many of those resources and references as I can recall.

(Note: As we attempted to pull this section together, and the footnotes included in the text, with Sandy's direction, we identified and included every reference we could find that she might have used. There were so many, as her research, books, articles, internet websites, were significant. If we have omitted any source that should have been included, we sincerely apologize to the source owner and will make every effort to correct the omission in any future publications.
—John)

There are so many website references and studies about MCS. It would be impossible to identify them all, but here are some that I found particularly helpful and informative:

https://www.multiplechemicalsensitivity.org

https://www.ewg.org/foodscores

http://www.chemicalsensitivityfoundation.org

https://eeoc.com/policy/laws/americans-with-disabilities-act-of-1990/

https://ourlittleplace.com

https://www.mcsfriends.org

There are other books and resources I want to share. Even if I did not reference them in the book, I have found them to be informative and helpful in my understanding of MCS.

Some books and other documents that have been helpful to me, include:

- Dr. Mercola online article: *7 Domestic Factors That Can Make or Break Your Health*

- *Multiple Chemical Sensitivity A Survival Guide* by Pamela Reed Gibson, MD

- *The Autoimmune Solution* by Amy Myers, MD

- *The Autoimmune Solution Cookbook* by Amy Myers, MD

- *The Thyroid Connection* by Amy Myers, MD

- *Home Safe Home* by Debra Lynn Dadd

- *The Daniel Plan Cookbook* by Rick Warren, Daniel Amen, MD and Mark Hyman, MD

- *The Complete Idiot's Guide to Thyroid Disease* by Dr. Alan Christianson and Hy Bender

- *Detoxify or Die* by Sherry A. Rogers, MD

- *Clean, Green and Lean* by Dr. Walter Crinnion

- *The Autoimmune Epidemic* by Donna Jackson Nakazawa

- Steinemann, Anne, PhD. "National Prevalence and Effects of Multiple Chemical Sensitivities" *Journal of Occupational and Environmental Medicine* 60: Issue 3, 152-156.

Appendix C
The Top Five Toxic Chemicals in Everyday Use

The following article is printed with permission. It was written by Jon D. Kaiser, M.D., and is available for download at: https://www.hopeforfatigue.org/cancer-fatigue-blog/the-top-5-toxic-chemicals-in-everyday-products.html

Chemicals in our everyday environment produce a toxic burden, which affects every system of our bodies right down to the mitochondria. Mitochondria make the energy our cells need to function properly. When mitochondria are exposed to environmental toxins, energy function fails and cells begin to die.

The high lipid content of mitochondrial membranes pull chemicals into the mitochondria like a magnet. This creates a disproportionate amount of these toxins inside the mitochondria. The higher or more frequent the exposure, the greater the likelihood of toxic effects occurring. The additive exposure to many of these chemicals coming from multiple sources spread out over decades is what is most alarming.

TOXIC CHEMICALS TO WATCH FOR

1. Plastics and Fragrances (Phthalates)

Phthalates are used to soften plastics and help bind chemicals and scents (fragrances) together. Phthalates affect mitochondrial activities by altering the permeability properties of the inner mitochondrial membrane and inhibiting key enzymatic processes.

These chemicals have been implicated in reproductive damage, depressed leukocyte function, and cancer. Phthalates have also been shown to impede blood coagulation, lower testosterone, and alter sexual development in children.

Phthalates are found in almost anything scented (shampoo, shaving lotion, nail polish, air fresheners, laundry detergent) cleaning products, insect repellent, carpeting, vinyl flooring, the coating on wires and cables, shower curtains, raincoats, plastic toys, and your car's steering wheel, dashboard, and gearshift. Medical devices are also full of phthalates – IV drip bags and tubing are made from phthalates to make them soft and pliable, effectively pumping them directly into the bloodstream of patients.

How to avoid phthalates:

Check plastic products: Plastic products with recycling codes 3 and 7 may contain phthalates or BPA. Look for plastic with recycling codes 1, 2, or 5. Whenever possible, avoid using plastic containers!

Avoid using plastic in the kitchen: Opt for glass food storage containers and choose bottles and sippy/snack cups that are made of stainless steel, silicone, or glass. Do not heat food in plastic containers, because the heat can accelerate the leaching of chemicals.

Shop wisely: Check your cosmetics and household products for the words, "fragrance" or "perfume" on a label which almost always means phthalates. Instead, look for items that say, "no synthetic fragrance" or "scented with only essential oils" or "phthalate-free."

2. Pesticides (OPs)

Organophosphates are one of the most toxic groups of substances used throughout the world. They are used in pesticides as well as biochemical weapons/agents.

Organophosphates target mitochondria and promote oxidative damage triggering cell death.

Organophosphates are also known as endocrine disruptors.

They affect complex hormonal processes that regulate growth, metabolism, fertility, and the immune system. OPs have also been linked to obesity, asthma, allergies, and cancer. Children exposed to organophosphates have more than twice the risk of developing pervasive developmental disorder (PDD), an autism spectrum disorder.

How to avoid organophosphates:

EAT ORGANIC FOOD: Avoid exposure to pesticides in your elimination of systemic toxins.

3. Plastics and Canned Foods (BPA)

Bisphenol A (BPA) is a plasticizer found in a wide variety of consumer products, including water bottles (recycle #7), canned foods, and in credit card and cash register receipts.

BPA is a strong mitochondrial toxin and has been linked to infertility, breast and reproductive system cancers, obesity, diabetes, and behavior changes. It has even been associated with resistance to chemotherapy treatment.

Manufacturers of baby bottles, sippy cups and sports water bottles switched to other plastics in 2009 upon mounting consumer pressure. Though the FDA banned BPA in baby bottles and children's cups in 2012, the FDA still allows BPA in food cans. Researchers at the Harvard School of Public Health determined that volunteers who ate a single serving of canned soup a day for five days had ten times the amount of BPA in their bodies as when they ate fresh soup daily.

How to avoid BPA:

Limit your intake of canned foods: Choose fresh or frozen foods.

Go for powdered versus liquid baby formula: The packaging of powdered formula contains less BPA. If

138

your baby needs liquid formula, look for brands sold in plastic or glass containers.

Check recycling labels: Favor plastic containers with recycling codes 1, 2, 5.

Reheat foods properly: Do not microwave food in plastic containers.

Say no to receipts: If you handle a receipt, wash your hands before preparing or eating food. Keep any receipts in an envelope. Do not allow children to hold or play with receipts.

4. Flame Retardants (PBDEs)

Brominated flame-retardants are used in various products to increase their resistance to fire and/or high temperatures.

Often found in televisions, computers, insulation, foam products, including children's toys and baby pillows, PBDEs have been shown to cause mitochondrial damage by increasing the production of free radicals. Exposure has been associated with neurotoxicity and thyroid conditions.

How to avoid PBDEs:

Know your materials: Look for products advertised as "free of flame retardant."

Avoid exposure: The foam in sofas and pillows may contain large amounts of PBDEs. Replace any furniture with exposed foam.

Rid your home of dust: Use a high-efficiency HEPA filter vacuum to clean up PBDE particles that have shed in dust around your house.

139

5. Antimicrobial Products (Triclosan)

Triclosan is an antimicrobial agent used in personal care products (soap, toothpastes, shampoos, hand and household sanitizers, etc.). It can even be infused into kitchen utensils.

Triclosan is a potent mitochondrial toxin. It interferes with muscle function disrupts hormone regulation and alters immune function. Triclosan's biggest danger is its possible contribution to the development of antibiotic-resistant germs, leading many companies to begin removing it from their products.

How to avoid triclosan:

Don't go antimicrobial: Avoid using hand soap and other household products labeled as "antibacterial."

Check ingredients; check labels for triclosan. While it's been said you can achieve "better living through chemistry," scientific research is revealing that many common household products contain chemicals that have toxic effects on our health. However, armed with the above knowledge and a growing number of "environmentally-friendly" products on the market, you can limit your exposure to these toxic chemicals, and protect yourself and your family from their health-damaging effects. Start by reducing your exposure to those that are most obvious.

Appendix D
WHAT CAN I DO TO PROTECT MYSELF AND THOSE AROUND ME?

If you have been fortunate enough to get this far in your life without experiencing any of the effects of the harmful chemicals that surround all of us, you should thank your Heavenly Father for this blessing.

But you are now aware of the MCS danger, and it is apparent that the danger for that and many other immune system diseases are growing exponentially (as a September 2020 article titled "Your 50+ Immune System" in the *AARP Bulletin* magazine reported). It was also reported that we are dealing with thousands of chemicals that were not in our environment 50 years ago, and others not even 20 years ago. These chemicals can and do alter immune function. As also reported in the article, The Centers for Disease Control and Prevention (CDC) has counted hundreds of environmental chemicals* that reach

*https://www.cdc.gov/biomonitoring/environmental_chemicals.html

measurable levels in our bodies, and we can clearly use some relief.

Here are some of the precautions you can take to protect yourself and those around you. You will note that most of these tips involve avoiding something, rather than buying or otherwise procuring some product to give you this protection.

First, here are some things you can do in your everyday life to protect yourself, especially if you have started to recognize some of the symptoms we have talked about in this book, or if you plan to be in the company of someone who suffers from MCS:

1.   Avoid coated cookware – use stainless steel pots and pans with glass tops.

2.   Use organic cotton sheets, washcloths, towels, and any other such items.

3.   Wash clothes that are not made from organic cotton several times before wearing, using Free and Clear soap, vinegar, and Borax before drying them and contaminating the dryer. Don't mix these special loads with other clothes.

4.   Eat only organic foods.

5.   Wash all fruit and vegetables before eating. Here are some tips to be sure you get it right, from the University of Maine Cooperative Extension Publication # 4336e:

   a.   Wash your hands with hot soapy water before and after preparing food.

b. Clean your countertop, cutting boards, and utensils after peeling produce and before cutting and chopping. Bacteria from the outside of raw produce can be transferred to the inside when it is cut or peeled. Wash kitchen surfaces and utensils with hot, soapy water after preparing each food item.

c. Do not wash produce with soaps or detergents.

d. Use clean potable cold water to wash items.

e. For produce with thick skin, use a vegetable brush to help wash away hard-to-remove microbes.

f. Produce with a lot of nooks and crannies, like cauliflower, broccoli or lettuce, should be soaked for 1 to 2 minutes in cold clean water.

g. Some produce, such as raspberries should not be soaked in water. Put fragile produce in a colander and spray it with distilled water.

h. After washing, dry with clean paper towel. This can remove more bacteria.

i. Eating on the run? Fill a spray bottle with distilled water and use it to wash apples and other fruits.

j. Don't forget that homegrown, farmers market, and grocery store fruits and vegetables should also be well washed.

k. Do not rewash packaged products labeled "ready-to-eat," "washed" or "triple washed."

l. Once cut or peeled, refrigerate as soon as possible at 40°F or below.

m. Do not purchase cut produce that is not refrigerated.

6. Avoid foods that have been grown with pesticides, and don't use pesticides in your home garden or lawn.

7. Avoid artificial fragrances – don't use them and avoid being around those who do.

8. Stay away from kerosene, gasoline, and other petroleum products.

9. Use glass containers for food storage.

10. Monitor the quality of air in your home and in your car. There are many air quality monitors available, including at Amazon.com with a wide price range. We used the IQAir Air Visual Pro which monitors PM2.5, CO2, AQI, Temperature and Humidity.

11. Change your auto's cabin filter regularly.

12. Wear a mask and avoid touching the door handle in public restrooms.

13. Use a water filtration system in your home.

14. Use fragrance-free hand wipes when in restaurants.

15. Wear a mask when driving in heavy traffic or near polluting factories.

16. Use water, vinegar, and baking soda instead of common household cleaners.

17. Replace toxic dishwashing solutions with Free and Clear products.

18. Clean your ovens, sinks, and drains with baking soda and vinegar.

19. Don't use mothballs.

20. Don't use dryer sheets.

21. Don't use plug-in air fresheners.

22. Avoid public places where heavy scents are likely to be worn.

23. When repairmen are coming to your home, advise them in advance of the requirements for entering.

If you are in the process of building a home or remodeling an existing one, these tips should be helpful. These are things we learned and applied to our new Blue Ridge Log Cabin in Tryon:

1. Proper ventilation throughout your home.

2. No gas furnaces or fireplaces.

3. Use paints that do not have lead in them, and do not move into a house that has lead-based paint in it.

4. No carpeting.

5. No particleboard in home construction.

6. No chemical spraying for insects.

7. Avoid any exhaust fumes in your home.

8. No attached garages to avoid fumes from gasoline.

9. Locate your home so it is not in the vicinity of toxic fumes.

Appendix E

Chemicals Can Cripple:

What you need to know before visiting a person who has MCS

Years ago, we identified a small booklet that explained our situation in easy-to-understand terms. We would email it to anyone who would be visiting us in our home, and if they would read it and heed the advice it contained, they would be well prepared for a rewarding visit.

We attempted to locate the author of this booklet, and after several searches found one place where it was attributed to Kathy Houghton. We were unable however, to locate Ms. Houghton, but located the following:

https://kathy-mcspage.blogspot.com/2007/03/visiting-person-who-has-mcs.html

This booklet may have been done in connection with https://multiplechemicalsensitivty.org.

We would like to express our sincere appreciation for all the help this small booklet provided us over the years.

The following is a paraphrased summary of the preparation requests we would send.

We wanted our visitors to understand that while we looked forward to seeing them, if they didn't follow these requirements, their visit could be a disaster. Their very presence could trigger terrible reactions in their host and result in a very short and unpleasant time together. Setting the stage in this way would usually go a long way toward getting their attention, resulting in a good faith attempt at compliance.

We explained that it wouldn't be about them as a person that would trigger my inability to breathe, watery eyes, and overall discomfort. It would be about any chemicals they had put on their body that was making it impossible for us to be together.

We pointed out that any product that included the word "scented" in its label would not be allowed in our home. Even things like mints, gum, or scented toothpaste won't work.

Specific details were given for products that were sure to cause a reaction:

- Shampoos – Don't even try to find one that works. I will provide you with what you need in advance of your visit. (We liked Bronner's liquid products)

- Soap – Same story, same solution. As you are traveling from your house to ours, you need to avoid

using the soap solutions found in public restrooms
along the way.

- Nail polish – Don't

- Deodorant – Don't use any or use a product like Arm
  and Hammer unscented.

- Hand creams and lotions – Best to just avoid their
  use during our visit.

- Clothing – I can't be around clothes that have
  been washed in any scented detergents or bleach.
  There are a number of Free and Clear products on
  the market, as manufacturers seem to be starting
  to understand. New clothes need to be washed a
  couple of times before that "new clothes smell" can
  be removed.

Even with detailed explanations and instructions,
we often would find that our visitors would enter
the house only to be told immediately that we had a
problem. Then they would reflect on their activities
and recall that they had applied nail polish last night,
used a commercial deodorant or shampoo or washed
their hands in that fast-food restaurant on the way over.

We were always aware of the difficulty getting
ready for a visit would cause our friends and loved
ones. The result, which was probably inevitable, was
that eventually we pretty much just stopped having
them. Even when family would visit, we would house
them in a local motel or B & B so we could avoid any
serious problems.

The preparations that we would have to insist on should be, to some degree, employed by everyone as they become proactive in their drive to avoid developing MCS.

Toxic products are harmful to everyone.

The only difference between an MCS sufferer and someone who has not yet begun having reactions to toxic products is that the sufferer knows immediately when they are in the presence of products that are harmful.

The non-sufferer, while in the presence of these products, just doesn't know it.

Yet.

9 781852 980146

CPSIA information can be obtained
at www.ICGtesting.com
Printed in the USA
FSHW021011081221
86696FS